The Gendering of Madness in Victorian and Modern England and America

The Gendering of Madness in Victorian and Modern England and America

The Gendering of Madness in Victorian and Modern England and America

By

Leslie Ann Harper

Cambridge Scholars
Publishing

The Gendering of Madness in Victorian and Modern England and America

By Leslie Ann Harper

This book first published 2024

Cambridge Scholars Publishing

Lady Stephenson Library, Newcastle upon Tyne, NE6 2PA, UK

British Library Cataloguing in Publication Data
A catalogue record for this book is available from the British Library

ISBN (10): 1-5275-5296-9
ISBN (13): 978-1-5275-5296-8

This book is dedicated to my grandparents,
Marjorie Jane Landers Brohm, who always spoke her mind,
and Richard Elmer Brohm, who always encouraged
my academic pursuits.

TABLE OF CONTENTS

LIST OF ILLUSTRATIONS

ACKNOWLEDGEMENTS

I would like to thank Dr. Suzette Henke and Dr. Annette Allen for their guidance and support throughout my doctoral program, as well as their guidance in writing and revising my dissertation. I would also like to thank Dr. Nancy Theriot for her patient and painstaking efforts to assist me improving this work. I also appreciate the advice of Dr. Mary Rosner regarding the chapter on *Lady Audley's Secret*, and I appreciate Dr. Glenn Crothers pointing me towards invaluable resources regarding the Mary Lincoln case.

This book would not have been possible without the help of many family members. First and foremost, I could not have completed this work if not for the support of my mother, Patricia French, who babysat countless times while I was researching and writing. I would also like to thank my father, Stephen French, as well as Michael and Karen Harper, Judy Brohm, Carl Reckelhoff, and Betty Overstreet for their voluntary babysitting services and support. Finally, I would like to thank my husband, Tim Harper, for supporting my decision to go to graduate school and for his understanding and patience. And last but not least, I am grateful for my children—Eli Patrick, Annabel Lee, and Madeline Jane Harper—for helping me to retain my own sanity by providing a never-ending source of light. I love you all.

INTRODUCTION

In her groundbreaking work *The Female Malady*, Elaine Showalter calls attention to the tendency to associate mental illness with women. For centuries there has been "an equation between femininity and insanity" (Showalter, *Female* 3). Many feminist scholars have noted this association and have developed various theories to explain it. Some scholars have argued that there are more cases of insanity in the female population because women have literally been driven mad by their social roles and limited opportunities in a patriarchal society. Others have interpreted "insane" behavior as the only means of protest available to women in a patriarchal society. Still others have argued that the label of "insanity" has been applied to rebellious women as a means of discipline and punishment. Regardless of the reason for this association between women and mental illness, the association is incontrovertibly present in Victorian and Modern England and America. According to Showalter, "By the middle of the nineteenth century, records showed that women had become the majority of patients in public lunatic asylums" (*Female* 3).

In the following study, I will examine the cultural association between women and madness by analyzing historical accounts, literature, and visual art from the Victorian and Modern periods. Theories and categories of mental illness in the nineteenth and early twentieth centuries both reflected and encouraged an association between women and madness that was prominent in Victorian and Modern culture. Likewise, the cultural association between women and madness is visible in the art of the nineteenth century, particularly through the pre-Raphaelite obsession with Ophelia. Historical accounts of women who were institutionalized as insane in the nineteenth century reveal how damaging this cultural association could be, as the label of "madness" was often applied for the sake of controlling women. Both the literary and historical accounts I examine demonstrate an awareness of how the label of "madness" could be used as a means of controlling women in Victorian society.

Madness is a slippery concept that changes over time and varies from culture to culture. As Michel Foucault explains, "mental illness has its reality and its value qua illness only within a culture that recognizes it as such" (60). Doctors create a variety of disease categories to differentiate between what they understand as different types of mental illness, but there is rarely consensus about diagnoses and treatments even among healthcare professionals living in the same time and place. Although categories of mental illness are culturally constructed and, therefore, fluid, different cultures do have a common method of diagnosing so-called insanity: "illness is defined in relation to an average, a norm, a 'pattern'" (Foucault 62).

Across cultures, therefore, madness is linked to deviancy from whatever a given society considers normal. As Stephen Trombley writes, "the insane are always *guilty*—of some transgression against society and the prevailing codes of that society" (210). Thus, the first insane asylums were built in the middle of the seventeenth century to house "all those who, in relation to the order of reason, morality, and society, showed signs of derangement" (Foucault 67). These first asylums were not places of treatment but places to intern those whom society wanted to exclude because of their deviation from the norm. Michel Foucault points out that when Pinel freed the "mad" of their physical chains at the end of the eighteenth century, "he reconstituted around them a whole network of moral chains" (71). As Foucault explains, "sanctions were immediately applied to any departure from normal behavior. All this took place under the direction of a doctor whose task was not so much that of therapeutic intervention as that of ethical supervision" (71). In the Victorian and early Modern periods, doctors continued this work of ethical supervision. Both the diagnosis and treatment of insanity during this time reveals "an attempt on the part of the medical profession to enforce unwritten social codes as if they were the law of the land" (Trombley 2). Medical doctors and men in general seem to have seen it as their duty to incarcerate and, sometimes, to rehabilitate deviants in order to preserve the purity of society.

In a patriarchal society, women are particularly vulnerable to being punished for deviancy from the accepted norm. Because of the cultural association between women and madness in Victorian and Modern England and America, women who rebelled against social conventions could be dismissed as "mad" and summarily punished with institutionalization or any number of medical "treatments" designed to enforce submission to social standards of appropriate behavior. Those who opposed the Women's Rights Movement often depicted advocates of the movement as mentally imbalanced, presumably for no other reason than that they were standing up for themselves and stepping outside of their prescribed gender role. The gendered construction of mental illness has allowed some women who were not mentally ill to be labeled as such. The women who wrote the asylum narratives I look at both claimed to be and seem perfectly sane in their testimony. However, they were non-conformists and that in and of itself was sufficient reason for being labeled mentally ill in their society.

Though much of this study focuses on how categories of mental illness are culturally constructed, I am not suggesting that mental illness does not exist. On the contrary, I believe that some people suffer from mind or mood problems that impair their ability to function. I offer Virginia Woolf and Charlotte Perkins Gilman as two examples of women who suffered from some form of mental illness. Woolf and Gilman believed they suffered from mental illness themselves and actually sought medical treatment, though they were critical of the treatment they received. Thus, all of the women I examine have one thing in common: they were all active protestors—not passive victims—in regard to how they were perceived and/or treated by the medical community.

Although the ways that women were perceived and treated in regard to mental illness in Victorian and Modern times was detrimental to their freedom and their sanity, women repeatedly refused to assume the role of passive victim that doctors and the patriarchy tried to force on them. To demonstrate this basic thesis, I have divided this book into eight chapters which make four different moves. In the first two chapters, I lay the foundation for the study by establishing the cultural association between women and madness in the Victorian and Modern periods. In chapters three and four I examine how this cultural association impacted historical cases of women who were labeled "mad" and placed in asylums. Chapters five and six are devoted to two literary representations of institutionalization that address how the label of "madness" could be used as a means of controlling women in Victorian society. The final two chapters are devoted to female authors who perceived themselves as suffering from mental illness but who protested the ways that they were treated by the medical community and society at large. While the authors of asylum narratives take a more direct approach in their protests and these latter women protested through more subtle fictional accounts, they all rejected the role of silent victim in actively voicing their discontent with diagnoses and treatments of mental illness.

In my first chapter, I explore how the experience and label of "mental illness" was gendered in the Victorian and Modern periods in America and England. I begin by discussing the methods of diagnosis and theories that nineteenth-century physicians used to explain symptoms of mental illness in women. I then provide an overview of several categories of mental illness that were associated with a particular gender, such as anorexia nervosa, nymphomania, kleptomania, puerperal insanity, hysteria, neurasthenia, shell-shock, and multiple personality disorder. Ultimately, this examination will reveal how medical science is embedded in the culture in which it is practiced and how it has been used to justify and enforce cultural values, particularly in regard to gender.

Chapter 2 examines the pre-Raphaelite obsession with Ophelia. Ophelia was the most popular subject in English art in the nineteenth century. During that period, at least fifty portraits of Ophelia appeared in exhibitions at the Royal Academy (Kiefer 12). The prominent role Ophelia played in nineteenth-century art is attributable to the fact that she personifies a stereotype of femininity that captivated the Victorians: the young madwoman. Pre-Raphaelite paintings of Ophelia clearly reflected the Victorian association between women and madness. However, they also strengthened this association through constant repetition.

Chapter 3 is devoted to the examination of asylum narratives. In nineteenth-century America, many female revolutionaries were labeled mad and locked in asylums. As one woman learned from bitter experience: "When for any reason a person is wanted put out of the way, insane hospitals stand with outstretched arms ready to embrace them" (Pennell 151). While some students of women's studies are familiar with the story of Elizabeth Packard, society at large is not. Moreover, there are dozens of stories like hers that have been all but forgotten. Although Geller and Harris have compiled a collection of such tales, these stories have not yet received the attention they deserve. Perhaps contemporary scholars do not realize how many true stories exist about rebellious women confined in madhouses. In the second half of the nineteenth century, however, many people were aware of this appalling epidemic. In her autobiography, Elizabeth Cady Stanton commented, "Could the dark secrets of insane asylums be brought to light we should be shocked to know the great number of rebellious wives, sisters, and daughters who are thus sacrificed to false customs and barbarous laws made by men for women" (214). In this chapter, I will resurrect the histories of some of those who have been buried alive in a madhouse and forgotten. An examination of these accounts reveals that these women were commonly imprisoned in asylums for boldly asserting their religious, economic, and domestic rights.

Various women in the nineteenth and early twentieth centuries were institutionalized for unconventional behavior and religious beliefs, but the most famous of these was Mary Lincoln, to whom I devote Chapter 4. In 1875 Mary Lincoln's only surviving son Robert had her tried for insanity and placed in an asylum. Soon afterwards, Mary began a campaign to free herself, insisting that she was the sane victim of a heartless son who had her institutionalized for selfish motives. Thus began the controversy surrounding Mary Lincoln's insanity case. While there is much debate among historians as to whether or not Mary Lincoln was truly insane, her contemporaries generally agreed that she was. She was a domineering, temperamental, quick-witted woman during a time when the world expected women to be silent, submissive, and supportive. Over the years, her unconventional behavior caused many people to question her sanity. However, the behavior that contributed most directly to her incarceration was connected to her excessive shopping and her Spiritualism.

The next two chapters address how asylums were portrayed in literature through inspections of *Lady Audley's Secret* and *The Woman in White*. Since the early eighteenth century, the English public was concerned about the danger that sane people were being confined in insane asylums. The Madhouse Act of 1774 tried to put an end to this concern by requiring a medical certification of insanity for each admitted patient. Despite this and subsequent reforms, wrongful incarcerations continued into the Victorian era, and public anxiety erupted in a series of lunacy panics. Several works of non-fiction were released by former inmates testifying to wrongful incarceration, and newspapers frequently "printed articles demanding inquiries and suggesting reforms" (McCandless 342). These tales inspired several sensational novels—Henry Cockton's *Valentine Vox* (1840), Wilkie Collins's *The Woman in White* (1860), and Charles Reade's *Hard Cash* (1863). I will devote a chapter to *The Woman in White*, analyzing how the novel's message about the wrongful institutionalization of women is undermined by the characterization of these women as being mentally unstable.

Although *Lady Audley's Secret* (1862) was also published shortly after an incarceration scare, critics have not traditionally examined the novel in this historical context. Critics interpret Lady Audley's institutionalization as a metaphor for the oppression of the disempowered Other who deviates from societal norms, and they laud the subversive nature of the novel. However, examining Braddon's book in relation to the lunacy panic drastically changes the way we understand the text. By her own admission, Braddon's book was a response to Wilkie Collins's *The Woman in White* (N. Donaldson vii), the sensational novel most commonly linked to the incarceration scare. While Collins's heroine is a frail, innocent woman in need of a savior, Braddon's is a dangerous woman who needs to be institutionalized for the safety of society. Both the depiction of Lady Audley's commitment and the motives of the characters in the novel indicate that Braddon's story is a reaction against the lunacy panic rather than another story fueling that panic. *Lady Audley's Secret* is not an exposé deploring the wrongful incarceration of social deviants. Braddon rather sympathizes with the doctors who try to protect society from such deviants. Braddon's response to the lunacy panic is likely influenced by the experiences of those close to her, specifically John Maxwell and Edward Bulwer-Lytton. Braddon lived with Maxwell for fourteen years and had five children with him before they could be married, as he already had a wife living in a mental institution. Due to her own situation, Braddon may have been sensitive about accusations regarding the wrongful institutionalization of family members. In addition, the novel was dedicated to her mentor and friend, Edward Bulwer-Lytton, a man who had his own wife incarcerated just a few years before the novel's publication.

The next chapter focuses on a writer who incorporated her experiences with mental illness and its treatment into her work—Charlotte Perkins Gilman. In both her 1935 autobiography and her 1892 short story "The Yellow Wallpaper," Gilman not only paints a graphic portrait of a woman suffering from mental illness, she also paints a vivid portrait of how such women are treated by the medical community. Importantly, Gilman's stated purpose in writing "The Yellow Wallpaper" was to protest the "rest cure" that she felt nearly drove her to "utter mental ruin" ("Why").

The last chapter is on Virginia Woolf. Like Charlotte Perkins Gilman, Virginia Woolf suffered from mental illness. She heard voices, had recurrent bouts of depression, suffered from delusions, and had disabling migraines. Despite all of these symptoms, Woolf often said there was nothing truly wrong with her and blamed herself for her own emotional problems and for the problems of those around her. During her depressive moods, Woolf sometimes felt as though she deserved to be punished, and she often refused to eat. Over the course of her life, Woolf had several breakdowns in which she went "mad" and had to seek medical treatment, and she attempted suicide twice unsuccessfully. While this mental disorder led to her eventual suicide in 1941, it also inspired some of the greatest novels of the twentieth century. Woolf was able to beautifully weave her own tragic experience with mental illness into her art. The character of Septimus Smith from *Mrs. Dalloway* and "The Prime Minister" is a strikingly poignant example of Woolf's ability to incorporate experiences from her own bouts of insanity into her work. Moreover, like Gilman, Woolf criticizes the attitudes and treatments of healthcare professionals in her literary depictions of physicians.

By exploring the medical theories, historical accounts, literature, and visual art of the Victorian and Modern periods, I hope to firmly establish the cultural association between women and madness in England and America. This book will contribute to the conversation by offering an interdisciplinary approach. I will incorporate the theories of philosopher Michel Foucault and literary scholar Elaine Showalter, as well as the work of medical historians like Carroll Smith-Rosenberg and Nancy Theriot. In addition, I will provide my own analysis of selected texts and artworks relating to madness from these periods. Finally, I will connect this work with the asylum narratives of Victorian and Modern women that have long been underappreciated. By doing so, I will reveal how damaging the cultural association between women and madness really was by giving historical examples of women who were negatively impacted by the association. More importantly, I will demonstrate that these women were not passive victims, but active protestors of the laws, diagnoses, and treatments that had a negative impact on their lives.

CHAPTER ONE

CATEGORIES OF MENTAL ILLNESS

In this chapter, I will explore how the experience and label of "mental illness" was gendered in the Victorian and Modern periods in America and England. I will begin by discussing the methods of diagnosis and theories that nineteenth-century physicians used to explain symptoms of mental illness in women. I will also provide an overview of several categories of mental illness that were associated with a particular gender, such as anorexia nervosa, nymphomania, kleptomania, puerperal insanity, hysteria, neurasthenia, shell-shock, and multiple personality disorder. Ultimately, this examination will reveal how medical science is embedded in the culture in which it is practiced and how it has been used to justify and enforce cultural values, particularly in regard to gender.

Until the end of the nineteenth century, physicians' diagnoses relied almost entirely on patient descriptions of illness. Doctors used the case method of taking the patient's medical history, family history, and symptoms. Not only were physicians supposed to note *all* symptoms, they were supposed to inquire into the patient's living conditions and circumstances leading up to the illness as well (Theriot, *Journal* 351). As Nancy Theriot explains, "patients and their families and friends came to physicians with physical and psychological symptoms; and physicians, also nineteenth-century men and women, defined these collections of strange behaviors and unaccountable physical ailments as specific diseases" (*Journal* 355). As Theriot suggests, doctors felt compelled to make a diagnosis and to "prescribe some course of action outside of the patient's self-care options in order to be considered a scientific practitioner" (*Journal* 356).

Many of the symptoms of "mental illness" that these patients—or more frequently, their families—reported were attitudes and behaviors that were not considered culturally appropriate. Unconventional behavior had been associated with mental illness since at least 1835, when Dr. James Cowles Prichard introduced the concept of "moral insanity" in England. This diagnosis "could be stretched to take in almost any kind of behavior regarded as abnormal or disruptive by community standards" (Showalter, *Female* 29). While moral insanity was a diagnosis of the Victorian period, its impact lasted into the modern era. In 1907, Dr. George Savage, one of the most renowned physicians of his day, defined insanity as "a disorder of mental balance which renders the person alien—that is, out of relationship with the surroundings into which he has been born, educated, and has hitherto fitted" (qtd. in Trombley 124). Similarly, Dr. Maurice Craig says in 1905 that "[i]nsanity means essentially then such a want of harmony between the individual and his social medium" (qtd. in Trombley 192). Of course, both Savage's and Craig's definitions of insanity underline the cultural embeddedness of the concept of mental illness. One is labeled "insane" if one does not conform to the ideas and behavior considered "normal" in one's society.

The identification of insanity with behavior and feelings that were deemed culturally inappropriate—especially for women—was embraced by the American and English public. Indeed, Theriot suggests that some diagnoses were created to satisfy the patients and families who came to doctors searching for explanations and cures for "insane" behavior. According to Theriot, family members typically brought women to physicians because of unwomanly behavior which they described as "insane." Importantly, "Most patients did not name their own behavior and feelings as nervous or insane; more frequently the connection was made by a family member or close friends" (Theriot, *Signs* 18). Husbands and mothers labeled their wives and daughters "mad" if they were contradictory, sexually promiscuous, or neglectful of their appearance. If a woman did not ascribe to the cult of true womanhood, she risked being dragged to the doctor's office for treatment for her "insanity." Thus, "The nervous symptoms and deviant behavior of nineteenth-century women patients were shaped by the constraints of gender and then were medicalized and therefore legitimized by medical representation as disease" (Theriot, *Signs* 24).

Confronted with explaining the assortment of symptoms their female patients presented, doctors fashioned a complex theory that connected seemingly unrelated symptoms to the female reproductive system and to femininity. The "reflex theory" of disease causation was the dominant explanation for women's illness in the latter half of the nineteenth century. Doctors posited that the female reproductive system was connected to the mind and all other parts of the body via the nervous system, and problems in one part of the body could cause problems in another seemingly remote area. Although there was a struggle among alienists, gynecologists, and neurologists for female patients in the nineteenth century, most physicians used the "reflex theory" to explain their ailments. Gynecologists "saw woman as the product and prisoner of her reproductive system" (Smith-Rosenberg and Rosenberg 335) and identified the uterus and ovaries as the cause of women's illnesses. Neurologists and alienists, on the other hand, identified the nervous system as the primary cause of women's illness: "In the neurological version of reflex, women's nervous and mental illness was rooted in a nervous system subjected to physical and/or situational stress" (Theriot, *Journal* 355). Physicians generally believed that heredity made someone predisposed to nervousness or mental illness, but alienists and neurologists argued that shocks to the nervous system through traumatic life experiences could trigger such illness. While they saw the nervous system as the primary conduit of illness in women, "most alienists and neurologists agreed with their gynecologist colleagues that women's reproductive organs dictated that women should restrict their activities and aspirations" (Theriot, *Signs* 9-10).

Victorian physicians argued that a woman only had a limited amount of energy, and that energy was required for the development of her uterus and ovaries. With the onset of puberty, therefore, a woman should retire from the public world. According to Carroll Smith-Rosenberg, "physicians routinely used this energy theory to sanction attacks upon any behavior they considered unfeminine; education, factory work, religious or charitable activities, indeed virtually any interests outside the home during puberty were deplored, as were any kind of sexual forwardness such as flirtations, dances and party-going" (*Feminist* 62). While women were discouraged from participating in any activity outside of the home, they were encouraged to do domestic chores as exercise. "Indeed, the life-style most frequently advocated for the young woman consisted of a routine of domestic tasks, such as bed-making, cooking, cleaning and child-tending" (Smith-Rosenberg, *Feminist* 62). Obviously, these medical prescriptions reinforced the Victorian ideology of "Separate Spheres." If a female did not obey these medical prescriptions/cultural guidelines, she would meet with dire consequences. Misbehavior could cause any number of problems: "She would become weak and nervous, perhaps sterile, or more commonly, and in a sense more dangerously for society, capable of bearing only sickly and neurotic children—children able to produce only feebler and more degenerate versions of themselves" (Smith-Rosenberg and Rosenberg 340).

Whereas behaving in an unladylike fashion was identified as a trigger—as well as a symptom—of mental illness, even adhering to appropriate standards of behavior was no guarantee of sanity. According to Smith-Rosenberg, "Menstruation, nineteenth-century physicians warned, drives some women temporarily insane; menstruating women might go berserk, destroying furniture, attacking family and strangers alike and even killing their infants" (*Feminist* 64). Although women were at risk of manifesting insanity during their menstruating years, they were also at risk after these years of menstruation were over. As Smith-Rosenberg explains, "nineteenth-century physicians used menopause as an all-purpose explanation for the heightened disease incidence of the older female; all of her ills were directly or indirectly diseases of the uterus and ovaries" (*Feminist* 65). Because of her precarious mental state, the menopausal woman, like the pubescent girl, was advised to avoid mental activities and busy herself with household chores (Smith-Rosenberg, *Feminist* 66). Thus, Victorian medical theories about women and illness re-enforced cultural norms about women's proper place in—or, rather, *out*—of society throughout their lives.

In 1896, one physician wrote that "women are especially subject to mental disturbances dependent upon their sexual nature at three different epochs of life: the period of puberty when the menstrual function is established, the childbearing period and the menopause" (qtd. in Theriot, *Women* 410). In other words, woman is vulnerable to insanity by virtue of her sex throughout her life. Given that the cultural association between women and insanity was concurrent with the association between insanity and unconventional behavior, it is not surprising that people were quick to apply the label of "mentally ill" to a woman who defied her culture's gender norms. No wonder families brought their disobedient wives and daughters to physicians for treatment. And no wonder that these disobedient women exhibited a variety of different, seemingly unrelated symptoms. As in any time and place, the English and American physicians in the Victorian and Modern eras created various disease categories to explain the collections of ailments that were presented to them.

One of the nervous disorders diagnosed in the Victorian era was anorexia nervosa. This disorder was identified in 1873 as an affliction troubling adolescent girls in England and France (Showalter, *Female* 127). In a report to the Clinical Society of London, Dr. William Whitney Gull described the major symptoms as emaciation, loss of appetite, amenorrhea, and restlessness. He attributed the disorder to a "morbid mental state," adding "it will be admitted that young women at the ages named are specially obnoxious to mental perversity" (qtd. in Showalter, *Female* 127). However, rather than disdaining the anorexic's unorthodox eating habits, some admired her martyrly behavior. In his essay on this neurosis, T. Clifford Allbutt praises the typical anorexic as an "unselfish" and "self-forgetful" young woman who appears too busy with her feminine duties to attend to her own health (qtd. in Showalter, *Female* 128). Anorexics had a particular aversion to meat, a phenomenon that Showalter explains by noting that "a carnivorous diet was associated with sexual promiscuity" (*Female* 129). Of course, Victorian women were not supposed to feel sexual desire. Thus, Showalter suggests that the Victorian anorexic was not attempting to defy cultural ideals about femininity but acting them out to an extreme degree. It is also possible that these girls were attempting to exert some small form of control over their own bodies in a society where they felt virtually powerless.

In their avoidance of meat, Victorian anorexics may have been trying to avoid another mental illness associated with women—nymphomania. Nymphomania was diagnosed as a disease of excessive sexual desire. Since Victorian women weren't supposed to feel sexual desire, those who expressed such feelings risked being labeled nymphomaniacs. Masturbation in particular was cited as both a symptom of nymphomania and a cause of insanity in women. Treatments for nymphomania included "injections of ice water into the rectum, introduction of ice into the vagina, and leeching of the labia and the cervix" (Showalter, *Female* 75). Sometimes surgery was prescribed: both the removal of the clitoris and the ovaries were accepted forms of treatment for nymphomania, as well as for other female ailments. The diagnosis of nymphomania reflects the Victorian fear of female sexuality, just as the treatments were a means of controlling it.

Nymphomania was one of several categories of mental illness that were associated with a diseased uterus. Dr. William Chapman Grigg, specialist in women's diseases at Queen Charlotte's Lying-In Hospital in London, wrote, "a disease of the upper portion of the uterus is a very common accompaniment of various forms of mania in women, such as melancholia, religious mania, nymphomania, and I have seen it in several cases of kleptomania" (qtd. in Abelson 130). Thus, a woman could be diagnosed as having one of a wide variety of disease categories that doctors associated with her reproductive system and, therefore, with her femininity.

Like many categories of mental illness that doctors eventually attributed to disease of the uterus, kleptomania was not gender specific when it initially appeared in 1840. However, by the time kleptomania became a widespread diagnosis in the 1870s, "the female reproductive economy . . . was understood to be the seat of the disorder" (Abelson 131). Not only was kleptomania gender specific, it was class specific as well. Elaine Abelson explains: "Stores lost merchandise from many sources—professional thieves, clerks, delivery men, and others—but only the middle-class female shoplifter was thought to be acting out of a medical disability" (124). In addition to shoplifting, the kleptomaniac's symptoms included headaches, nervousness, menstrual problems, and memory loss (Abelson 130). When a middle-class, female shoplifter claimed to suffer from this collection of symptoms, her "legal and moral innocence . . . were taken for granted by professionals and the public alike" (Abelson 124). Although middle-class women could utilize this disease category to excuse criminal behavior, it reinforced the belief that a woman's reproductive system made her susceptible to mental illness. Thus, this disease category could be exploited by one class of women, but it also strengthened the harmful cultural association between mental illness and women in general.

Another type of insanity that women in Victorian England and America were diagnosed with was puerperal insanity, a common ailment occurring in women during or after pregnancy. This type of insanity could take manic or melancholic forms. Prominent symptoms included talking incessantly, complaining of being wronged, obscene language, refusal to eat, homicidal tendencies toward husband and/or infant, suicidal tendencies, insomnia, constant weeping, and tearing off clothes. Some of these symptoms, along with the context in which they occurred, indicate that these women may have been rebelling against their gender role. However, "To nineteenth-century men, a woman who rejected her child, neglected her household duties, expressed no care for her personal appearance, and frequently spoke in obscenities had to be 'insane'" (Theriot, *Women* 409). Some women who suffered from puerperal insanity were treated at home; others were sent to rest homes and asylums. Indeed, puerperal insanity was listed as the cause for at least ten percent of asylum admissions (Theriot, *Women* 405).

Treatments for puerperal insanity included drug-induced sleep and the "rest cure" made famous by American physician Silas Weir Mitchell. Mitchell had his patients stay in a rest home where they were suspended from all activity and contact with loved ones between six weeks and two months. While there, they were fed by nurses, whether they wanted to eat or not, and in many cases Mitchell "arrange[d] to have the bowels and water passed while lying down" (*Fat* 59). During this period of suspended activity, he expected his patients to gain about fifty pounds (Appignanesi 120). Sometimes he would let patients read for an hour or two a day, but never more than three. Doctors and nurses sometimes used a device to masturbate patients, making the day "less tiresome than might be supposed" (Mitchell, *Fat* 6). While some women attested that the "rest cure"—a treatment for various illnesses that afflicted the nerves—truly did cure them, others disagreed. Charlotte Perkins Gilman wrote "The Yellow Wallpaper" to demonstrate how Mitchell's "rest cure" nearly drove her mad. Beginning in the 1890s, the diagnosis of puerperal insanity began to be out of vogue and women lost this disease category as a possible sick role, as its different manifestations were subsumed under the broader categories of mania or melancholy (Theriot, *Women* 413).

Undoubtedly the most famous female malady is hysteria. The identification of hysteria as a woman's illness is evident in its very name;

"hysteria" is derived from the Greek word for womb (Showalter, *Female* 129). The ancient Greeks believed that the uterus "was a free-floating entity which could leave its moorings when a woman was dissatisfied, to travel around the body and disrupt everything in its passage" (Appignanesi 142). Similarly, the "reflex theory" allowed Victorian physicians to attribute "virtually every known human ill" to hysteria (Smith-Rosenberg, *Social* 662). While some doctors diagnosed men with hysteria as well, by far the majority of hysterical patients were women. According to Showalter, rebellious young women were particularly susceptible to this diagnosis (*Female* 145).

Like hysteria, neurasthenia could be blamed for a wide variety of seemingly unrelated symptoms. When George Beard identified neurasthenia as "the morbid condition of the exhaustion of the nervous system" in 1869 (qtd. in Appignanesi 101), he listed over fifty symptoms, including "fainting, tooth decay, irascibility, paralysis, lack of appetite, vomiting, fits of laughing and crying, neuralgia, muscle spasms, morbid fears, constipation, insomnia, weariness" (Appignanesi 115). Most of these were also symptoms of hysteria. Indeed, the two maladies shared so many symptoms that they were virtually indistinguishable even to specialists (Showalter, *Female* 134). Pierre Janet, one of the pre-eminent experts on hysteria, suggested that neurasthenia was just a more prestigious name for hysteria that American physicians used to diagnose their patients "for the [sake of the] family" (11). The difference between the two illnesses seems to revolve around class. Showalter claims that neurasthenics were "ladylike, and well-bred" (*Female* 134). Although doctors diagnosed members of both sexes with neurasthenia, it was a much more common diagnosis for women than men (Russett 118). Women were thought to be naturally more nervous than men and, therefore, more prone to nervous exhaustion (Russett 118). Of course, Victorian scientists also argued that women needed their energy for reproduction, and any extra energy spent on intellectual pursuits—or anything else outside of the domestic sphere—would drive them to nervous exhaustion.

While neurasthenia may have become a diagnosis for members of the upper class who suffered from hysterical symptoms, shell-shock became the diagnosis for men suffering from hysterical symptoms in the modern age of warfare. As Judith Herman explains, "Under conditions of unremitting exposure to the horrors of trench warfare, men began to break down in shocking numbers. Confined and rendered helpless, subjected to constant threat of annihilation, and forced to witness the mutilation and death of their comrades without any hope of reprieve, many men began to act like hysterical women" (20). During World War I, over twenty army hospitals had to be hastily set-up to treat soldiers suffering from mental breakdowns (Showalter, *Female* 168-69). After the war, 114,600 ex-soldiers applied for pensions for shell-shock (Showalter, *Female* 190). According to one estimate, shell-shock accounted for 40 percent of British casualties (Herman 20). Although these men suffered hysterical symptoms, their malady was labeled "shell-shock." As Elaine Showalter explains, "The efficacy of the term 'shell shock' lay in its power to provide a masculine-sounding substitute for the effeminate associations of 'hysteria' and to disguise the troubling parallels between male war neurosis and the female nervous disorders epidemic before the war" (*Female* 172). Despite the macho name, military officials and doctors generally treated victims of shell-shock with disdain, dismissing them as effeminate. Showalter explains, "madness, even when experienced by men, is metaphorically and symbolically represented as feminine: a female malady" (*Female* 4). Doctors like Lewis Yealland "treated" victims by shaming them and torturing them with electric shock. In contrast, W. H. R. Rivers used talk therapy to heal patients (Showalter, *Female* 176-78).[1] In 1941, after nearly twenty years of working with war veterans, American psychiatrist Abram Kardiner published *The Traumatic Neuroses of War*, in which he recognized shell-shock as a form of hysteria (Herman 23-24).

Another category of mental illness associated with hysteria in the Victorian and Modern periods was multiple personality disorder (MPD). Physicians in various western countries discovered that when hysterics were placed under hypnosis, alternate personalities could appear. Although the earliest known cases of MPD occurred in 1791, MPD was reported with increasing frequency towards the end of the following century (Crabtree 288, 301). In an article published in 1887, Pierre Janet theorized that "this kind of doubling of personality was at the very heart of the hysterical condition" (qtd. in Crabtree 310). Janet believed that subconscious personalities formed around memories that the patient could not cope with, and that they "affect the perceptions, emotions, and actions of the individual in such a way that the normal personality feels at odds with himself or herself, subject to phobias, compulsions, hallucinations, and other symptoms for which there is no apparent explanation" (Crabtree 320). Janet provided many examples of MPD in hysterics, as did Sigmund Freud and Joseph Breuer. Breuer's treatment of Bertha Pappenheim, also known as "Anna O.," became the model for the "talking cure" of psychoanalysis. In America,

---

[1] Rivers "held to Freudian concepts of the unconscious and repression to explain the process by which moments of terror or disgust were suppressed and converted into physical symptoms" (Showalter, *Female* 189).

Morton Prince's study of the hysterical Miss Beauchamp (1898-1904) is one of the earliest and most famous studies of MPD.[2]

Not only do concepts of "mental illness" reflect the gender dynamics of a particular time and place, they also reflect race and class dynamics as well. Categories of "mental illness" like neurasthenia and hysteria were not just coded as female maladies; they were coded as maladies of *white* women. According to Michele Birnbaum, Victorian physicians believed that "women of color . . . lacked the extreme feminine sensibility and degree of cultural refinement" marking women who suffered from hysteria and neurasthenia (8). Laura Briggs also concludes that "The medical and scientific literature contained not only a portrait of the white, upper-class neurasthenic woman, but also a fully articulated counter-account of the impossibility of hysteria in rural, immigrant, non-white, and 'savage' women" (258). In their attention to race, both Birnbaum and Briggs seem to amalgamate hysteria and neurasthenia together as one illness, when they became separated by class. As already discussed, neurasthenia seems to have developed a more positive connotation associated with the upper class than hysteria did.

Because disease categories like hysteria and neurasthenia were typically diagnoses reserved for middle- and upper-class white women, members of other sociological groups were excluded from these disease categories even when they exhibited the same symptoms. "It is only a covert romanticism," Carroll Smith-Rosenberg writes, that hysteria did not afflict the lower classes (*Social* 659). According to Mark Micale, new studies in Scotland and France indicate that "hysteria among the lower classes was not in fact rare before the nineteenth century, but simply unrecognized, untreated, and unreported" (157). Of course, hysteria was "unrecognized, untreated, and unreported" in the lower classes precisely because of the

---

[2] Miss Beauchamp came to Prince complaining of hysterical symptoms: headaches, insomnia, bodily pains, persistent fatigue, sleepwalking, nightmares, trances (Appignanesi172). While undergoing hypnosis, Miss Beauchamp revealed three alternate personalities. Prince characterized her waking self as "the Saint" (selfless, patient, polite, charitable), and the other personalities as Sally (mischievous, irresponsible, flirtatious, tomboy) and the Woman ("a parody of the New Woman who thinks she is 'capable of running the world'") (Appignanesi 173). Eventually Prince discovers that the original personality was not the Saint, but the Woman. The appearance of her male caretaker illuminated by lightening at her bedroom window literally scared Miss Beauchamp out of her mind. Her real self dissociated, and the Saint took over. As treatment, Prince integrated these two personalities and eradicated Sally (Appignanesi 171-76).

class connotations of the illness. Just as some members of the lower classes suffered from hysterical symptoms, some non-whites suffered from them as well. After spending 1843-1844 inquiring into "the diseases of the colored population of the South and West," Dr. Daniel Drake concluded that hysteria occurred "with considerable frequency" in the slave population (341-42). Evidently, Dr. Drake's colleagues had neglected to inform him that "It was absurd to expect that a Southern black should suffer from nervous diseases, or that insanity, epilepsy, and neurasthenia should flourish on the banks of the Amazon or the Nile" (Showalter, *Female* 135).

As Nancy Theriot points out, disease categories of past eras disappear not because they were not "real" to begin with, but because methods of diagnosis change (*Journal* 352). Moreover, concepts of disease are always shaped by culture and change over time. Victorian and modern theories of illness, disease categories, and methods of treatment depended on the symptoms described by the patient and/or her family, as well as the specialty of the consulting physician. There was undoubtedly debate regarding what constituted "mental illness" and how it was treated in Victorian and Modern England and America. However, an examination of the dominant theories, categories, and treatments for "insanity" in these periods reveals that medical science reinforced cultural values, particularly in regard to gender.

CHAPTER TWO

THE MAD MAIDEN IN THE MEADOW: DEPICTIONS OF OPHELIA IN PRE-RAPHAELITE ART

The association between women and madness that is evident in categories of mental illness in the nineteenth century is reflected in the art of the period as well. The depiction of one figure in particular helped perpetuate stereotypes about mental illness in women: Ophelia. Ophelia was the most popular subject in English art in the nineteenth century. During that period, at least fifty portraits of Ophelia appeared in exhibitions at the Royal Academy (Kiefer 12). Moreover, she was also the subject of poetry and photography. According to Kaara Peterson, portrayals of Ophelia in art changed dramatically around mid-century. Prior to this, whenever Ophelia was represented in art, she was typically part of a group and not the focus of the piece. After mid-century, however, she suddenly became the focal point as "the drowning, pathos-inspiring figure that typically haunts our imaginations today" (Peterson). Why were the Victorians—particularly the Pre-Raphaelites—so captivated by the figure of Ophelia? The prominent role Ophelia played in Pre-Raphaelite art is attributable to the fact that she combined two of the most fascinating female stereotypes in the Victorian imagination: the madwoman and the tragic youth.

An examination of nineteenth-century culture reveals that the Victorians were fascinated by the figure of the madwoman. She appears again and again in works of art, literature, and medicine throughout the period. The Victorians believed that madness was linked to a woman's physiology, and Ophelia is a prime example of this. "She is an especially intriguing character," Carol Kiefer writes, "because of her madness—a madness that is intimately linked to her femininity" (11).

In the nineteenth century, Ophelia becomes representative of madwomen in general. In fact, the character of Ophelia was a model for conceptions of female insanity in nineteenth-century medicine. According to Elaine Showalter,

> superintendents of Victorian lunatic asylums were also enthusiasts of Shakespeare, who turned to his dramas for models of mental aberrations that could be applied to their clinical practice. The case study of Ophelia was one that seemed particularly useful as an account of hysteria or mental breakdown in adolescence, a period of sexual instability which the Victorians regarded as risky for women's mental health. (*Shakespeare* 85)

Helen Small argues that both medical historians and literary critics have "produced an overly synthetic account of English fictional and medical representations of madness in the 18th and 19th centuries" (28). However, an examination of nineteenth-century medical texts reveals that this connection between madwomen in literature and medical texts was first made by nineteenth-century doctors themselves. John Charles Bucknill, the president of the Medico-Psychological Association, said in 1859: "Ophelia is the very type of a class of cases by no means uncommon. Every medical physician of moderately extensive experience must have seen many Ophelias" (qtd. in Showalter, *Shakespeare* 86). Likewise, Dr. John Connolly, superintendent of the Hanwell Asylum, believed that even the lay person could recognize the Ophelia type in a mental ward: "the same young years, the same faded beauty, the same fantastic dress and interrupted song" (qtd. in Showalter, *Shakespeare* 86). These same characteristics of madness are conveyed in the iconography of Pre-Raphaelite portrayals of Ophelia: "her appearance, her gestures, her costume, her props, are freighted with emblematic significance" (Showalter, *Shakespeare* 80).

Because Ophelia was both the victim of madness and the victim of rejected love, and because her suffering led to her early death, she is a conglomeration of the most tragic romantic fantasies of the Victorian age. As Bram Dijkstra explains, Ophelia became a perverse sort of idol, "the later nineteenth-century's all-time favorite example of the love-crazed self-sacrificial woman who most perfectly demonstrated her devotion to man by descending into madness . . . and who in the end committed herself to a watery grave, thereby fulfilling the nineteenth-century male's fondest fantasies of feminine dependency" (42). Male artists in particular were obsessed with the figure of Ophelia, as she embodied the male fantasy of the lovesick, fragile, dependent woman. For them, Ophelia's identity was defined by her status as Hamlet's spurned lover. The appropriate destiny for a rejected woman in Victorian art was an early death (Marsh, *Images* 139). As Jan Marsh explains in *Pre-Raphaelite Women: Images of Femininity*, representations of Ophelia belong to a larger class of paintings which Marsh calls the "Pale Ladies of Death." Although she was not the only female figure in Pre-Raphaelite art to represent "sorrowful, pathetic death" (Marsh, *Images* 138), Ophelia was certainly the most prominent.

The image of the dying maiden had a certain sex appeal for the Victorian male. As Gudrun Brokoph-Mauch explains, "The *femme fragile* is . . . the ideal playmate in the fantasy world of the sexually inhibited" (471). As a symbol of youthful innocence and fragility, the dying maiden is not sexually threatening. However, she is alluring to the male viewer precisely because she is "on the verge of sexual awakening" (Ziegler 41). Her early death, however, prevents that awakening and preserves her virginity. For this reason, Alan Young suggests that Ophelia's death symbolizes the containment of a threatening female sexuality (282). However, because her sexual innocence intensifies her sexual appeal, some Pre-Raphaelite illustrations of Ophelia are erotic. Jan Marsh explains: "Death, love and sex were powerfully but invisibly linked in Victorian culture and, as the century progressed, painters and poets made the link increasingly, even sensationally, explicit" (*Images* 135).

Because her tragic and sexual appeal is predicated upon her untimely death, most Pre-Raphaelite portraits of Ophelia illustrate her drowning or the moments just prior. Kaara Peterson blames the artistic repetition of Ophelia's death scene on Gertrude, the character who relates the tale of Ophelia's tragic end in the play: "Gertrude 'frames' Ophelia's story by making it as 'pretty as a picture,' and as such Gertrude's story becomes in turn the visual 'history' of the body of Ophelia, more often than not, as is evidenced by the artistic repetitions of this particular scene" (Peterson). Peterson is perturbed that "this one aspect of her life (death) has become essentially her entire story through a kind of synecdochic process—the part represents the whole." Gertrude's narrative of Ophelia's death is undoubtedly poetic and, therefore, a likely inspiration for later artists who took up the subject. However, this suggests that the figure of the maiden who dies of a broken heart was already a romantic icon in Shakespeare's time, just as it was for the Pre-Raphaelites. Moreover, Gertrude's poetic description of Ophelia's death may not be the only reason that she is typically portrayed in nature; perhaps Ophelia's placement in the wild is another allusion to her madness and, by extension, to woman's primitive nature.

The most famous representation of Ophelia does, indeed, illustrate her drowning in the wild. John Everett Millais's 1852 portrait of Ophelia captures the moment just before she sinks to her watery grave (see Fig. 2-1). Submerged in the stream, her arms are spread up in an attitude of surrender, reflecting the proper, passive female role. Her white dress symbolizes her virtue, while her flowing hair and anesthetized facial expression suggest her mental disarray. In one hand she grasps a trail of flowers, which floats alongside her in the stream. Both the flowers and the water are symbolic of the feminine and are, therefore, fitting surroundings for the death of a young maiden.

The story surrounding Millais's famous painting indicates just how pervasive the role of the submissive female martyr was in Victorian times. Millais's model for Ophelia was Elizabeth Siddal, a favorite of the Pre-Raphaelite Brotherhood. Although Millais painted the scenery on location outdoors, he painted Siddal in his studio in a tub filled with water. There were candles lit beneath the tub to keep the water warm, but when they went out Millais didn't notice. Siddal lay in the cold water silently, afraid to voice her discomfort for fear of disturbing the artist's concentration. As a result of lying in cold water for a prolonged period of time, Siddal became ill. In fact, forever afterwards she was to have health problems until her own untimely death. Siddal can thus be read as a living example of the Ophelia type, a woman who "placed the Pre-Raphaelites' work far above her own needs. She was a willing martyr to the cause" (Hawksley 43). Her submission to the male artists is again evident in her agreeing soon after this incident to Dante Rossetti's request that she not no longer model for other artists, as "he could no longer abide the thought of sharing her" (Hawksley 45). Although she was largely responsible for contributing to her family's income and such an arrangement would surely compromise her economically, Siddal obligingly agreed.

The same year that Millais's portrait of *Ophelia* appeared at the Royal Academy, Arthur Hughes exhibited a portrait of the same name (see Fig. 2-2). Unlike Millais, Hughes did not capture the drowning scene. However, Ophelia's imminent death is still present for the viewer familiar with her story, as Hughes portrays her perched on a tree just above the water. Furthermore, the frame is engraved with the lines from *Hamlet* where Gertrude describes how Ophelia "fell into the weeping brook" (IV.vii.174). As in Millais's piece, Ophelia is wearing a white dress symbolizing her purity. Her pale skin indicates illness, while her "emaciated form is suggestive of insanity" (Marsh, *Images* 138). Showalter describes Hughes's *Ophelia* as a "juxtaposition of childlike femininity and Christian martyrdom" (*Shakespeare* 85). Indeed, her crown of reeds is suggestive of Christ's crown of thorns, but she has the diminutive, elfish appearance of a child. This childlike appearance is reinforced by her behavior—scattering flowers in the stream before her. As in the play and the painting by Millais, Ophelia's association with flowers and a watery death are indicative of her fragile femininity.

Ophelia was the subject of Hughes's first Pre-Raphaelite work, and she was a figure he would return to again and again. Hughes painted a reduced oil replica of the original 1852 painting, as well as "a watercolour version of an unspecified Ophelia design" (Roberts and Evans 33). He also did two studies for a later painting, which appeared in the 1860s (see Fig. 2-3). Leonard Roberts and Mary Virginia Evans complain:

> Unlike in the 1852 Ophelia, which in her childlike innocence, her sense of abandonment, and uncomprehending attitude is a near-literal realization of Gertrude's description, the lady of the later version appears considerably older, and possesses a maturity of stature and poise inconsistent with either Hughes's first or Shakespeare's original Ophelia. (27)

It is true that the Ophelia of the earlier portrait is more childlike, though Gertrude's description of Ophelia does not particularly call to mind the image of a child. While Hughes emphasized Ophelia's childlike innocence in the first picture, in the second he preferred to emphasize her sexual appeal. Still youthful in appearance and draped in virginal white, the Ophelia of the later version is, nevertheless, undeniably more sensual, as indicated by her arm posed above her head, her naked shoulder, and her direct gaze at the viewer. Despite these changes, Ophelia retains the crown of reeds that recall Christ's martyrdom, and the flowers in her arms and hair once again emphasize her femininity. Although her flowing hair is, again, indicative of some kind of instability, it is not unkempt as it was in the previous portrait. Moreover, her downcast expression is more indicative of melancholia than insanity. Thus, the Ophelia of the later portrait more clearly evokes the image of the youthful maiden who dies of a broken heart. This was clearly Hughes's intention, as indicated by the lines from *Hamlet* that Hughes wrote on a label on the back of the painting. This time Hughes's portrait of Ophelia was inspired by her own words, as she mourns the loss of her father (*Hamlet* IV.5.188-98).[1] While Hughes, once again, does not show the moment Ophelia drowns, he does allude to it by having her veil trail towards the brook she walks beside.

Although they were not as well-known as the works by Millais and Hughes, Dante Gabriel Rossetti produced at least four different illustrations of Ophelia. In the first, an engraving done in 1858, Rossetti presents the

[1] Roberts and Evans note that these were the lines that "appear in Hughes's hand on a label on the back of the [second] painting" (28), but they fail to comprehend their significance, only complaining that Ophelia was insane at the time of this speech and she doesn't look insane in the portrait.

scene from Hamlet in which Hamlet spurns his lover (see Fig. 2-4). The frame emphasizes Hamlet's rejection of Ophelia, as it is inscribed with the lines: "I loved you not . . . Get thee to a nunnery" (Marsh, *Images* 138). Rossetti used himself as a model for Hamlet, while his betrothed—Elizabeth Siddal—was the model for Ophelia. As Jan Marsh explains, "There was bitter irony in Rossetti's choice of this scene from Hamlet, for in 1858 he apparently broke off his unofficial engagement to Lizzie" (*Images* 139). Like the broken-hearted Ophelia, Lizzie's rejection was the cause of her broken heart and her eventual death. Marsh recounts how "Lizzie vanished from view; there are no contemporary references to her in Pre-Raphaelite sources until 1860, when she reappeared on the scene, now seriously ill" (*Images* 139).

The parallel fates of Ophelia and Lizzie are reflected again in Rossetti's later portraits of Ophelia. In his 1864 portrayal, we see an Ophelia weakened in mind and body by the rejection of her lover (see Fig. 2-5). This frail female must lean upon her brother for support. This image of Ophelia may have been inspired by Lizzie's appearance when she "was gravely ill and, he believed, on the verge of death" after his rejection (Marsh, *Images* 141). Rossetti's sense of guilt prompted him to marry Siddal in an attempt to save her life. Rossetti seems to have interpreted a parallel sense of guilt in Hamlet, as his 1866 portrait of the lovers is an illustration of Hamlet kissing Ophelia's hand (see Fig. 2-6). Like Ophelia, however, Lizzie was already too ill to be saved. In her depression, she had developed an addiction to laudanum, and she died of an overdose in 1862. Perhaps Rossetti was reflecting on how his rejection of Lizzie had led to her mental imbalance and eventual death when he created his last image of Ophelia, the only one which is an allusion to her death scene (see Fig. 2-7). Rossetti's images show the progression of Ophelia's deterioration, possibly because he saw the parallels between her fate and Lizzie's. While the story of Ophelia must have held a personal significance to him, his representations of her nevertheless embody the archetype of the fragile girl who dies of a broken heart.

Another Pre-Raphaelite artist who used his wife as a model for Ophelia was George Frederick Watts. Watts was married to the actress Ellen Terry, who played the role of Ophelia on the stage. Terry actually visited a mental ward to study the role of the madwoman, but she discovered to her frustration that real madwomen were "too *theatrical*" to be of any assistance (qtd. in Showalter, *Shakespeare* 85). As Showalter explains, "This was because the iconography of the romantic Ophelia had begun to infiltrate reality, to define a style for mad young women seeking to express and communicate their distress" (*Shakespeare* 85). In Watts's 1864 painting of

Ophelia, Terry presents a subdued form of madness (see Fig. 2-8). Her pale skin and unkempt hair are signs of insanity common in the iconography of the madwoman but barely perceptible to the untrained eye.

After the portrait of Millais, the most famous visual representations of Ophelia are those of John William Waterhouse. His first portrait of Ophelia makes no allusions to her watery death but focuses instead on her insanity and sensuality (see Fig. 2-9). Jan Marsh describes the Ophelia of the 1889 portrait as “lying in a riverside meadow in an attitude of deranged abandon” (*Images* 140). The position of the body and the tousled hair are indicative of both sensuality and mental instability. Nevertheless, her white dress and position among the flowers suggests that she is still pure. The Ophelia of Waterhouse’s 1894 portrait has a similar sensuality, due again to the positioning of her body (see Fig. 2-10). Her hands caress her hair, as she seems to be lost in reverie. Like the earlier Ophelia, though, the 1894 version wears a virginal white. Her femininity is emphasized by the flowers and the lily pond, which, of course, alludes to her impending death. Waterhouse’s 1910 painting of Ophelia gives a slightly different representation than his other two pictures of the tragic heroine, though it still conforms to the iconography (see Fig. 2-11). In this illustration, Waterhouse seems to gravitate more to the figure of the madwoman than to the sensual maiden. The positioning of Ophelia’s body here is not sensual but hunched forward as if in distress. This sense of distress is further accentuated by her hands, which do not caress her hair. Instead, one hand grasps at the tree for support while another clings to her flowers and her dress. The most troubling feature of this Ophelia, however, is the wild look in her eyes as she stares directly at the viewer. Waterhouse has exchanged the white dress for a blue one, though blue also symbolizes purity due to its association with the Virgin Mary. Because of her deranged attitude and her placement near the lily pond, this Ophelia is representative of both the madwoman and the dying maiden, though she is not as overtly sensual as Waterhouse’s previous representations.

Although Ophelia was more commonly represented in the works of male artists than female, some women did take up this tragic figure. One of these women was the photographer Julia Cameron. According to Jan Marsh and Pamela Nunn, “novice photographers up and down the country . . . tried to imitate painterly Pre-Raphaelitism in photography” (93). Julia Cameron, however, is the best-known photographer associated with the movement, and she was no amateur. She joined the Photographic Society of Great Britain in 1864, she registered her pictures with the Fine Arts Register, and she exhibited her work in several different countries (Marsh and Nunn 93). She knew several of the Pre-Raphaelites—including Holman

Hunt, Rossetti, Millais, and Watts—and she drew her inspiration from similar subjects. Between 1867 and 1874, Cameron dedicated her art to capturing images from Shakespeare's plays, including several of Ophelia.

In an article on Cameron's Shakespearean subjects, Melissa Parlin argues that Cameron's "photographic characters transcended Victorian gender views by defying convention and asserting their independence" (30). Parlin claims that Cameron's photographs of Ophelia are "in direct contrast with nineteenth-century depictions that focus on her madness and suicide. Cameron's Ophelia is strong, thoughtful and vibrant, facing her circumstances, and sometimes viewers, boldly" (Parlin 41). However, it seems like Parlin's assessment of Cameron's photography is based on a combination of wishful thinking and ignorance of the Ophelia iconography. It is true, as Parlin claims, that Cameron does not depict the scene of Ophelia's death. However, as this chapter has shown, this scene is absent in many other nineteenth-century depictions of Ophelia. Of the Pre-Raphaelites, only Millais actually shows Ophelia in the water, and Hughes, Watts, Rossetti, and Waterhouse each created at least one painting of Ophelia in which the water is barely visible or altogether absent. Moreover, these artists employ some of the same characteristics in their depictions of Ophelia that Cameron does, though Parlin claims that Cameron rebels against the iconography through these very same tropes.

Cameron's first *Ophelia* photograph from 1867 shows a side profile of a woman looking into the distance (see Fig. 2-12). As in many of the Pre-Raphaelite representations of Ophelia, this figure seems preoccupied. Additionally, her hair is down, and she wears the flowers associated with Ophelia. Yet Parlin argues: "This photograph lacks most overtly Ophelia-like qualities of nineteenth-century portrayals" simply because she is not drowning or "deranged" (36). However, as Ellen Terry's comment about real madwomen being "too *theatrical!*" suggests, the Ophelia figure was rarely represented as deranged. Instead, she is typically seen as melancholy or lost in thought, as in Cameron's second 1867 photograph (see Fig. 2-13). Yet Parlin references this "contemplative" gaze as a way that Cameron defies conventional Ophelia iconography (36). Cameron's 1874 photographs of Ophelia are more indicative of mental instability than the melancholic 1867 portrayals (see Fig. 2-14 and Fig. 2-15). The Ophelia in these portraits has her hands in her unkempt hair as she does in the Waterhouse paintings. Though this gesture is indicative of insanity in the Ophelia iconography, Parlin suggests it symbolizes dissatisfaction and defiance in Cameron's photos (37). Similarly, Parlin interprets the direct gaze—which is indicative of insanity in Ophelia portraits by Waterhouse and Hughes—as an indication of defiance and mental clarity (35). Though

Parlin clearly wants to interpret Julia Cameron as defying the conventions of the Pre-Raphaelite Brotherhood, her photographs of Ophelia use the same iconography of the madwoman.

Ophelia is also represented in the poetry of at least two of the women associated with the Pre-Raphaelite movement: Elizabeth Siddal and Christina Rossetti. As Sandra Donaldson suggests, the narrative voice and imagery of Siddal's "A Year and a Day" is reminiscent of Ophelia, the role which she modeled for both Millais and Rossetti. Like Ophelia, the narrator laments the loss of her lover:

> Slow days have passed that make a year,
> Slow hours that make a day,
> Since I could take my first dear love
> And kiss him the old way (Siddal 1-4).

Like both Ophelia and Siddal, her lover's rejection has caused her health to deteriorate: "I lie among the tall green grass / That bends above my head / And covers up my wasted face" (Siddal 7-9). Moreover, her mind seems to have deteriorated as well: "Dim phantoms of an unknown ill / Float through my tired brain" (Siddal 13-14). In the end, only death by drowning offers relief from suffering:

> The river ever running down
> Between its grassy bed . . .
> Shall bring to me a sadder dream
> When this sad dream is dead. (Siddal 31-36)

Sandra Donaldson argues that "dead love became the focus of the fantasy which Siddal finally enacted in suicide" (130). Her reenactment of Ophelia's fate indicates just how detrimental the romantic archetype of the melancholy maiden dying of a broken heart could be to Victorian women.

Elizabeth Siddal was not the only woman to embrace this archetype. As Jan Marsh explains, "Poems which to modern ears seem morbidly to welcome youthful death were popular in the Victorian era and especially common in the work of Lizzie's sister-in-law Christina Rossetti" (*Elizabeth* 30). Rossetti's poem "Sleeping at Last" is another example of a poem that idealizes death. The narrator yearns to be "Sleeping at last, the trouble and tumult over, / Sleeping at last, the struggle and horror past" (Rossetti 1-2). Specifically, she wants to escape the pain of life through death, "Cold and white, out of sight of friend and of lover" (Rossetti 3). The female figure of the poem lies "Under the purple thyme and the purple clover" (Rossetti 10), evoking images of Ophelia. In addition to the voice of the melancholy lover, her yearning for death, and the imagery reminiscent of Ophelia, the repetition of the phrase "at last," could be a reference to Siddal's poem "At Last" (Faraci 8). Mary Faraci suggests, "Remembering Elizabeth Siddal as *Ophelia*, Rossetti honors the sister-in-law who served Millais's interpretation of Ophelia" (Faraci 8).

Ophelia was obviously a source of fascination for the Victorians. She combined the archetype of the madwoman with that of the young maiden who dies of a broken heart. However, as Elizabeth Siddal's untimely death illustrates, this image was not a healthy role model for young women to idealize. Unfortunately, Siddal was not the only woman captivated by this image. Helena Faucit Martin, a nineteenth-century actress, wrote: "Ophelia was one of the pet dreams of my girlhood—partly, perhaps, from the mystery of her madness" (qtd. in Ziegler 41). Moreover, Thomas Miller's poem "Reading Shakespeare," published in the 1836 women's annual *Friendship's Offering*, recounts how young women idealize the dying Ophelia. And men weren't the only people representing Ophelia as a figure to idolize. Anna Jameson's *Characteristics of Women, Moral, Poetical, and Historical*—published in London in 1832—holds up Ophelia as a role model for women to follow. With such romanticizing of this tragic figure, one must wonder how many other Elizabeth Siddals followed Ophelia to an early grave. Even women who did not look up to Ophelia as a role model could certainly have been harmed by her prominence in nineteenth-century art. Although Pre-Raphaelite paintings of Ophelia reflect the association between women and mental illness that already existed within the culture, they also strengthened that association through constant repetition.

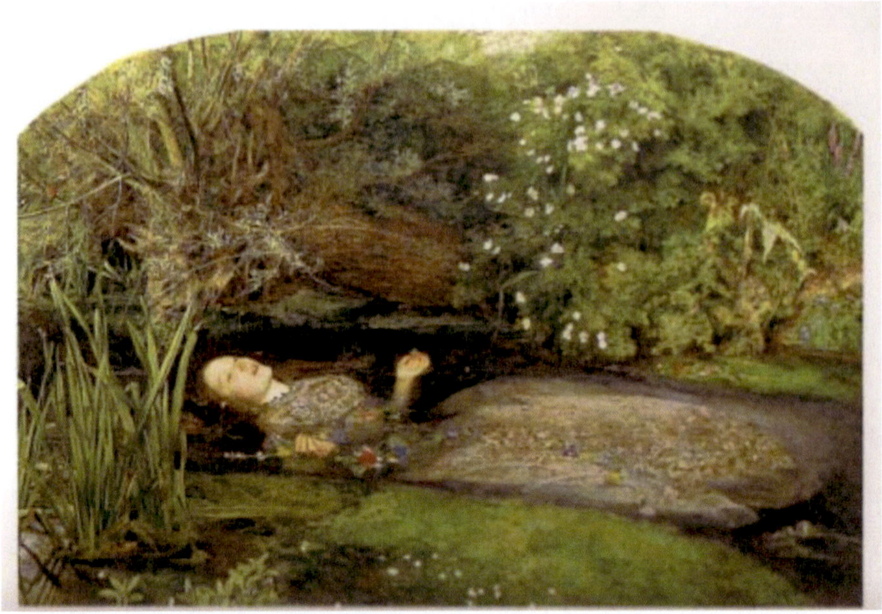

Fig. 2-1. John Everett Millais, *Ophelia,* 1851-52.

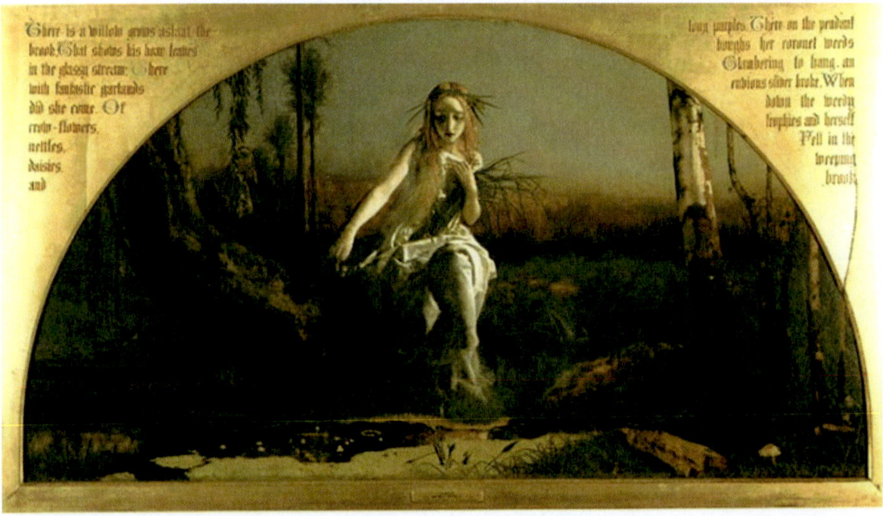

Fig. 2-2. Arthur Hughes, *Ophelia*, 1852.

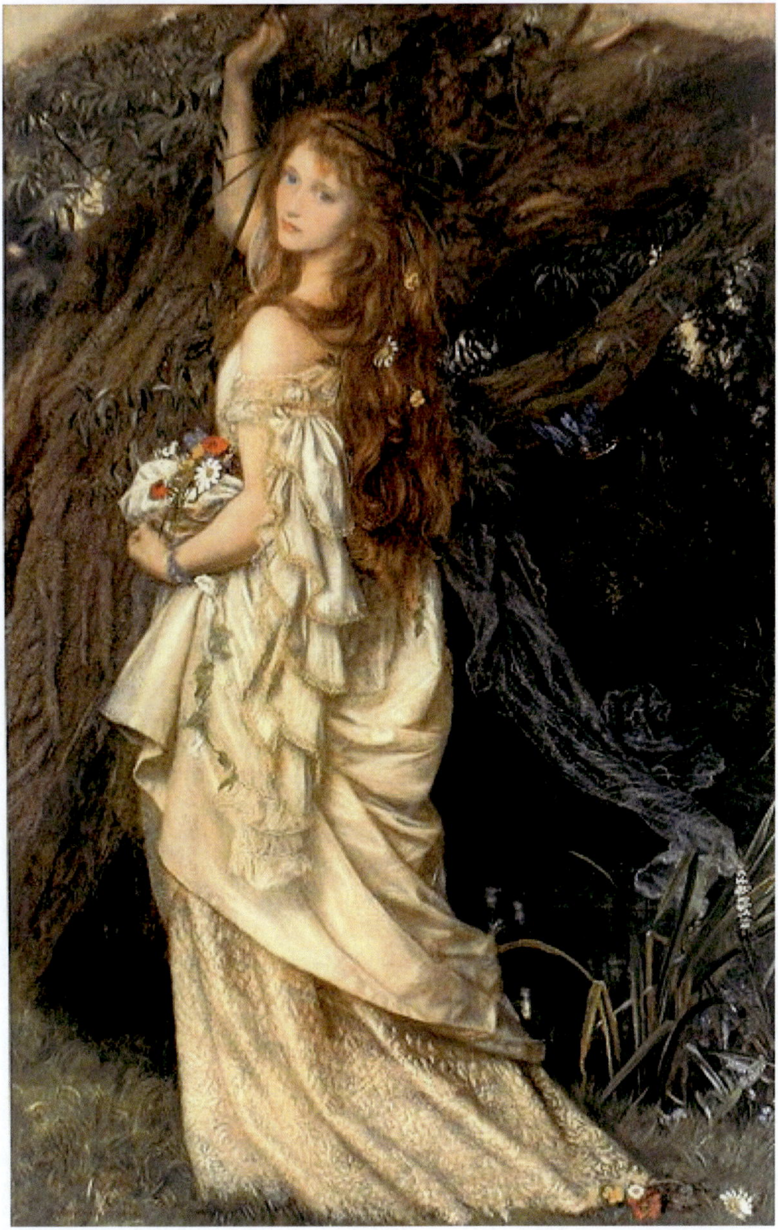

Fig. 2-3. Arthur Hughes, *Ophelia*, Circa 1865.

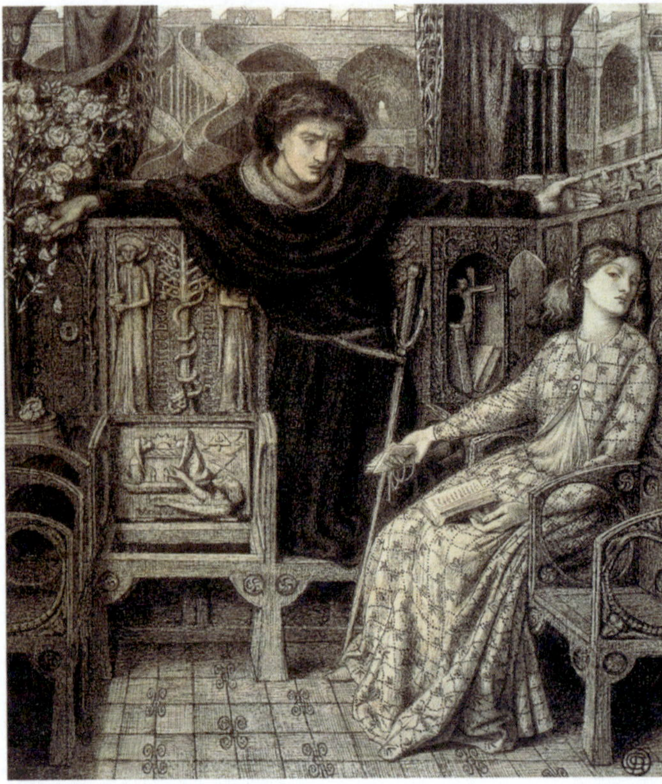

Fig. 2-4. Dante Gabriel Rossetti, *Ophelia Returning Hamlet's Betrothal Gifts*, 1858.

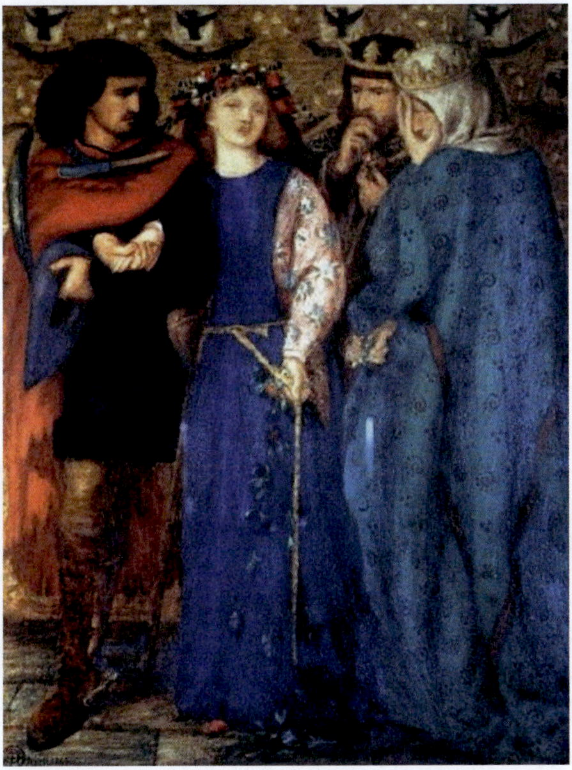

Fig. 2-5. Dante Gabriel Rossetti, *The First Madness of Ophelia*, 1864.

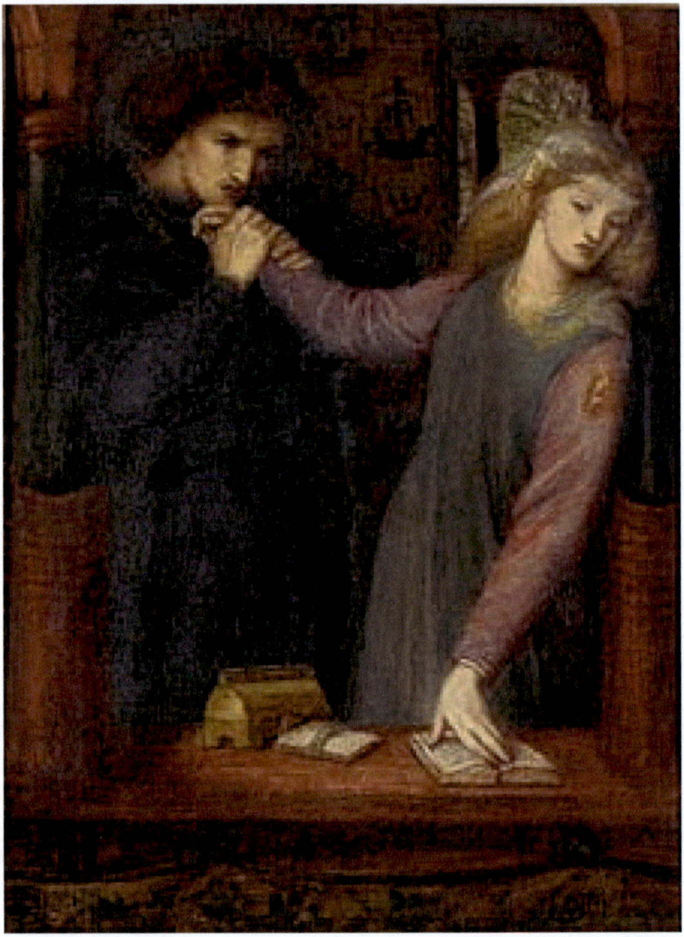

Fig. 2-6. Dante Gabriel Rossetti, *Hamlet and Ophelia*, 1866.

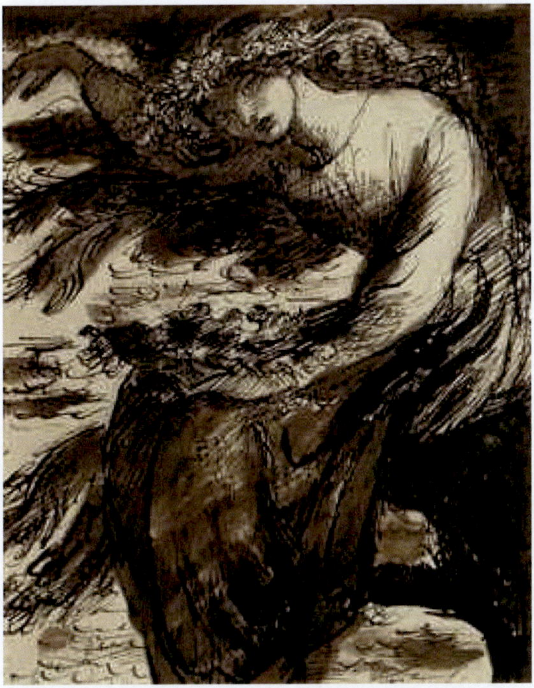

Fig. 2-7. Dante Gabriel Rossetti, *Ophelia*, 1870-75.

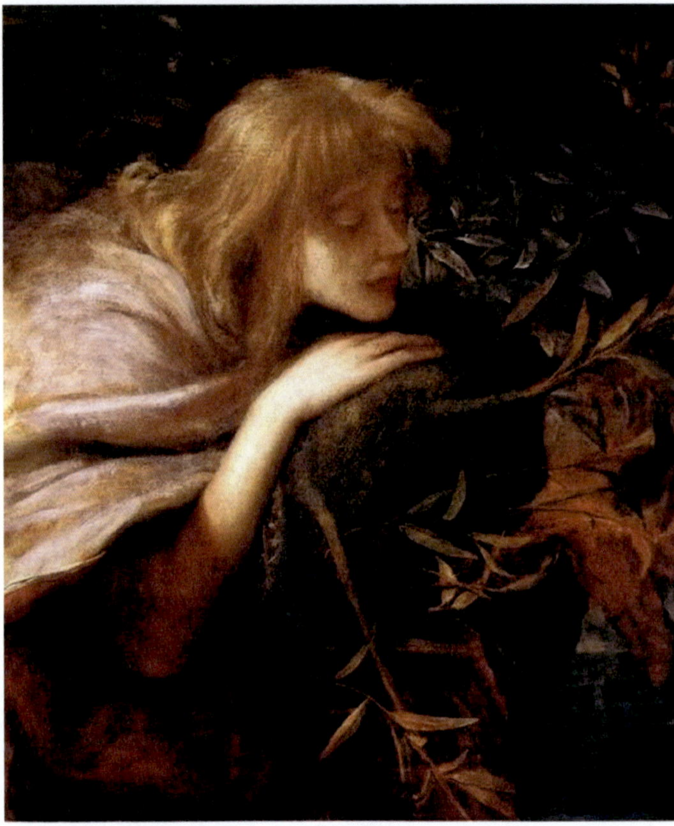

Fig. 2-8. George Frederic Watts, *Ophelia*, 1864.

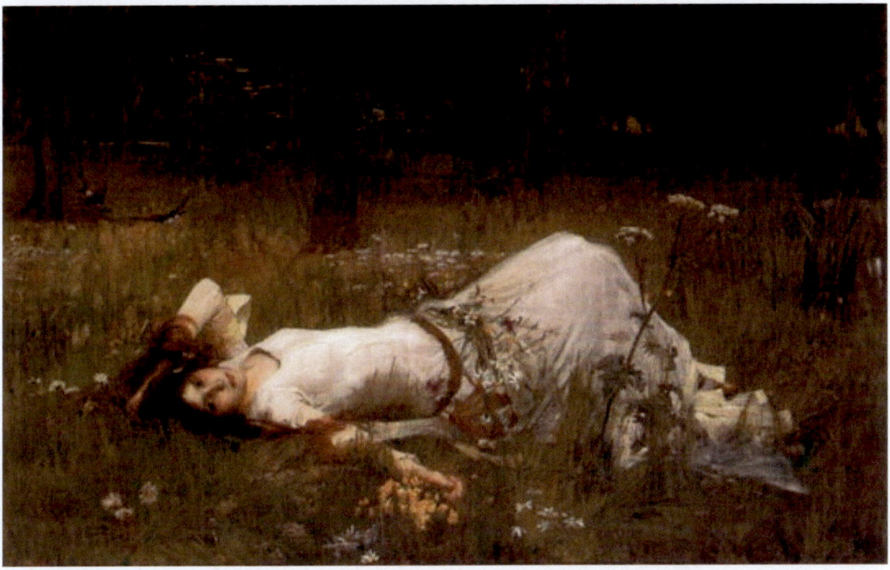

Fig. 2-9. John William Waterhouse, *Ophelia*, 1889.

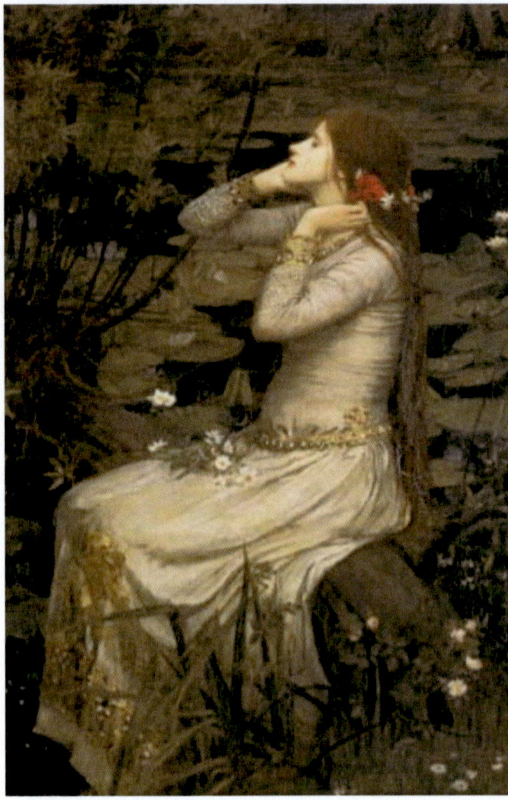

Fig. 2-10. John William Waterhouse, *Ophelia*, 1894.

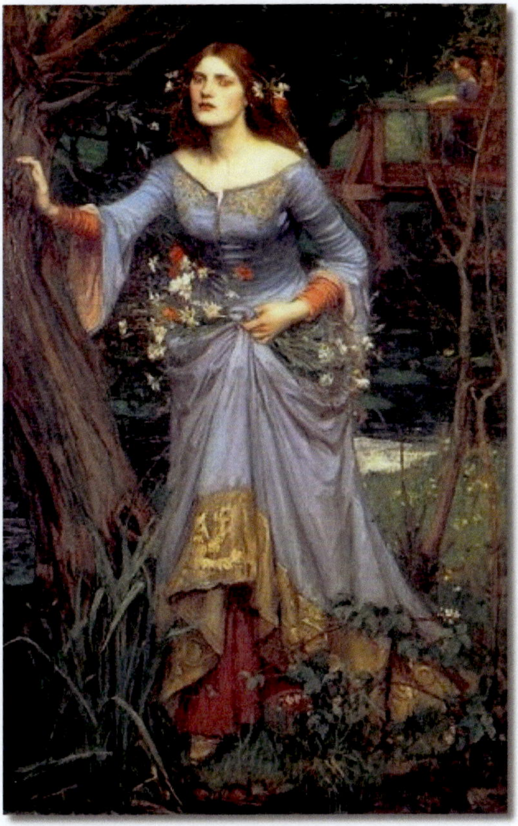

Fig. 2-11. John William Waterhouse, *Ophelia*, 1910.

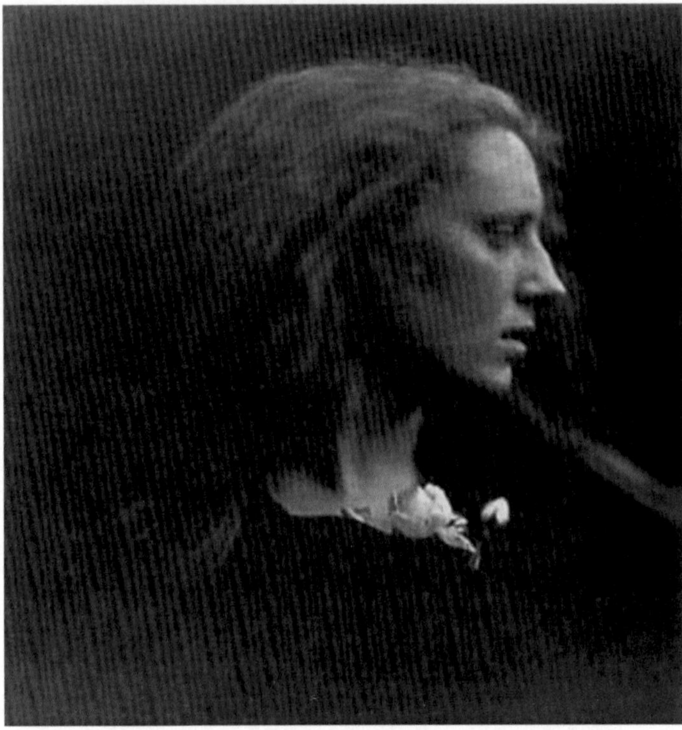

Fig. 2-12. Julia Margaret Cameron, *Ophelia,* 1867.

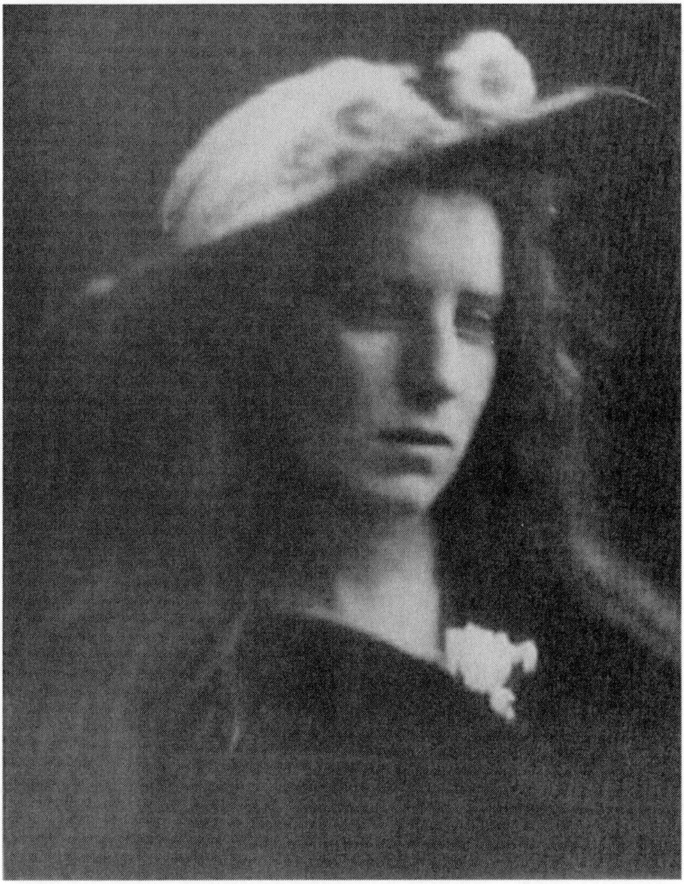

Fig. 2-13. Julia Margaret Cameron, *Ophelia Study No. 2*, 1867.

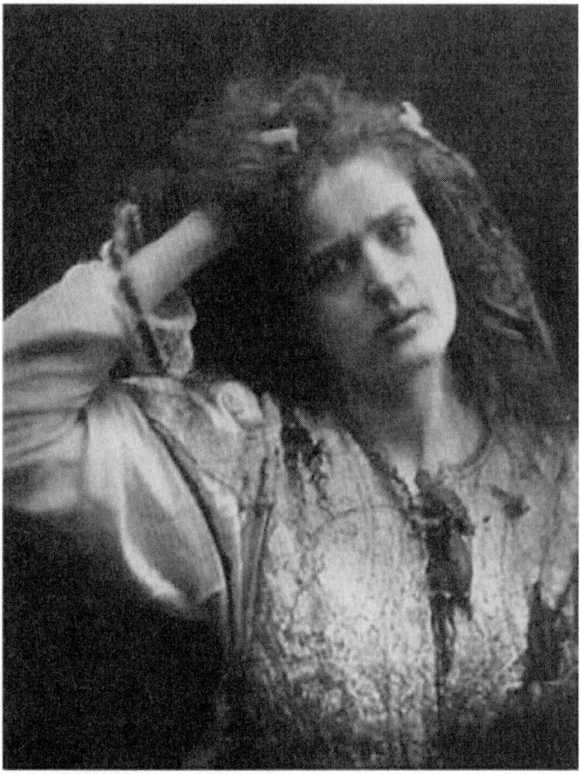

Fig. 2-14. Julia Margaret, *Ophelia*, 1874.

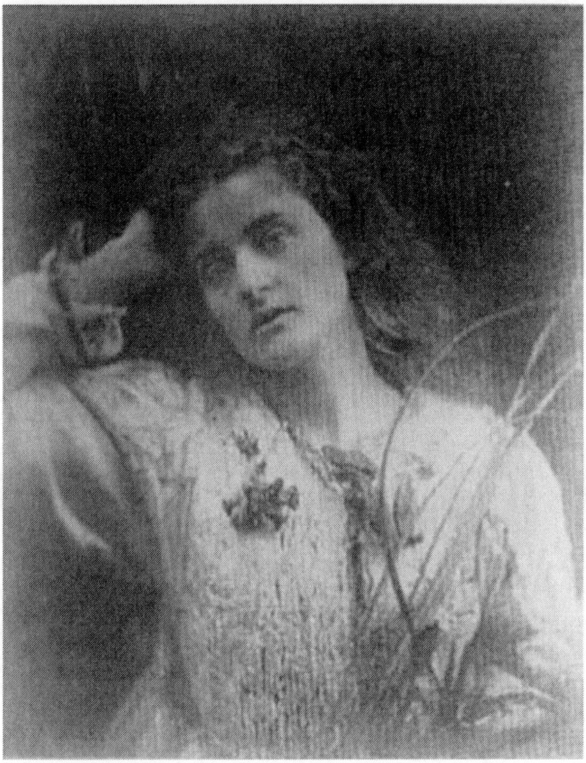

Fig. 2-15. Julia Margaret Cameron, *Ophelia,* 1874.

CHAPTER THREE

NO COUNTRY FOR BOLD WOMEN: INSTITUTIONALIZATION IN NINETEENTH-CENTURY AMERICA

The association between women and madness in Victorian culture had serious ramifications for some women. In nineteenth-century America, female non-conformists were particularly prone to being labeled "mad" given the belief that unconventional behavior could be attributed to mental illness and the cultural association between women and madness. As one woman learned from bitter experience: "When for any reason a person is wanted put out of the way, insane hospitals stand with outstretched arms ready to embrace them" (Pennell 151). Elaine Showalter identifies the label of "madness" as a typical form of punishment for transgressive women: "madness has been the historical label applied to female protest and revolution" (*Female* 5). In nineteenth-century America, many female revolutionaries were labeled "mad" and locked in asylums. While some students of women's studies are familiar with the story of Elizabeth Packard, society at large is not. Moreover, there are dozens of stories like hers that have been all but forgotten. Although Geller and Harris have compiled a collection of such tales, these stories have not yet received the attention they deserve. Perhaps contemporary scholars do not realize how many cases exist of bold women confined in madhouses. In the second half of the nineteenth century, however, many people were aware of this appalling epidemic. In her autobiography, Elizabeth Cady Stanton commented, "Could the dark secrets of insane asylums be brought to light we should be shocked to know the great number of rebellious wives, sisters, and daughters who are thus sacrificed to false customs and barbarous laws made by men for women" (214). In this chapter, I will resurrect the histories of some of those women who have been buried alive in a madhouse and forgotten. An examination of these accounts reveals that many of these women were imprisoned in asylums for boldly asserting their religious, economic, and domestic rights.

When these women stood up for themselves, they not only incurred the wrath of the men who sought to control them, they connected themselves to a larger movement for gender equality that was taking shape in nineteenth-century America. The first Woman's Rights Convention took place in upstate New York in 1848, and it was during this time leading up to the Civil War that female reformers began writing articles, giving speeches, and calling meetings on the subject of woman's rights. Historian Sylvia Hoffert argues that woman's rights advocates established their own discourse in which to protest their grievances and sway public opinion in their favor. They employed the language of natural rights because "it allowed them to place their demands within the respected and familiar American political tradition that had been established through the Declaration of Independence," and because it allowed them to expose the hypocrisy of those who wished to deny such rights to women (Hoffert 40)[1]. In addition to employing the language of John Locke, "One of the metaphors that woman's rights advocates frequently used to describe the general condition of women and to force the American public to address the issue of gender equality in the public sphere was one that suggested that women were no better than slaves" (Hoffert 55).[2] An examination of asylum narratives reveals both the same emphasis on natural rights as well as references to women as slaves. While early feminists also "tended to refer to society, its institutions, and the prejudices which limited opportunities for women, as a confining physical enclosure" (Hoffert 57), such references were not metaphorical in asylum narratives. Rather, the asylum narratives dramatically illustrate how confined women could be in nineteenth-century America, particularly when they tried to declare their rights.

Perhaps the most famous case of unjust institutionalization in nineteenth-century America was that of Elizabeth Packard, a woman who was punished for asserting her religious rights. Elizabeth left behind detailed—and numerous—accounts of her persecution. By all accounts, Theophilus and Elizabeth Packard shared a happy marriage for twenty years before problems arose. However, in the winter of 1859 they began to argue

---

[1] In fact, in the Declaration of Sentiments released at the 1848 Convention, "woman's rights advocates appropriated the language of the Declaration of Independence and changed very little of it" (Hoffert 40).

[2] This rhetorical strategy was already employed by eighteenth-century feminists like Mary Wolstonecraft and Mary Astell. "This rhetorical tradition, combined with the fact that . . . many early woman's rights were directly and deeply influenced by the abolitionist movement, provided them with a frame of reference from which to protest the status of women as well as a powerful metaphor to express their discontent" (Hoffert 56).

over religion. Theophilus was a Calvinist preacher, and Elizabeth had begun to question Calvinist doctrines. Elizabeth believed neither in the inherent depravity of man nor the doctrine of predestination. Moreover, she believed slavery to be a sin and felt a moral obligation to combat it. Disturbed by his wife's opinions and her increasing loquacity on the subject (she had voiced her beliefs in Bible study), Theophilus began to tell people that she was insane. Elizabeth's public withdrawal from her husband's church and subsequent attendance at a Methodist house of worship seemed to confirm her insanity for members of her husband's congregation.

Although Elizabeth was only "trying to enforce the First Amendment on behalf of women" (Chesler xviii), she soon found out that women in America were not afforded religious rights. While Elizabeth Packard was preparing for her morning bath on June 18, 1860, two physicians—both members of her husband's congregation—and the town sheriff arrived to escort her to an insane asylum. As Elizabeth made a hurried attempt to dress herself, her husband broke into the room with an axe. The doctors felt her pulse and, without further ado, promptly pronounced Elizabeth Packard to be insane. When she refused to go to the asylum without a trial allowing her to defend herself against the charge of insanity, her husband informed her that the laws of Illinois afforded her no such protection. The testament of two doctors and the resolve of the husband was all that was required to commit a woman to an asylum. Once in the asylum, Elizabeth Packard could not be released without the consent of her husband, who refused to do so unless she recanted her religious beliefs. Packard remained confined in the asylum for three years, when her eldest son came of age and persuaded his father to release his mother into his custody. After her release, she stayed with the family of her adopted sister for four months before returning home to her husband and children. However, after her return Mr. Packard locked his wife in her room and barred all communications with the outside world. After discovering that she was about to be sent to another insane asylum for life, Elizabeth passed a letter through the slit in her window to a man walking by. He delivered the letter to a friend of Elizabeth's, who sought help from a judge. The judge advised the friend to gather witnesses for a writ of *habeas corpus*, and Mr. Packard was ordered to bring his wife to court for a trial.

The purpose of the trial—which took place January 11th to the 19th, 1864—was to determine whether Elizabeth Packard was sane and, therefore, unlawfully imprisoned. Witnesses testifying for Mr. Packard claimed that Mrs. Packard was sane in all issues except religion. One of the original physicians who committed her testified, "I thought her partially deranged on religious matters. . . . On all other subjects she was perfectly rational" (Packard, *Marital* 20-21). The other physician found her to be insane primarily because of her aversion to certain Calvinist doctrines and her belief that she was in the right and her husband was in the wrong (*Marital* 23). While the Superintendent of the Illinois State Hospital that admitted Packard did not testify, he sent a letter stating that "Three-fourths of the religious community are insane in the same manner, in my opinion. . . . I would say that she is insane, the same as I would say Henry Ward Beecher, Spurgeon, Horace Greely, and like persons, are insane" (*Marital* 19). Mr. Packard's sister and her husband testified that Elizabeth was insane on the subject of religion, as did other member of the congregation. Like the doctors testifying for Mr. Packard, these witnesses believed Elizabeth to be insane only because she disagreed with them on points of theology. While this seemed to be sufficient reason to condemn Elizabeth amongst her husband's congregation, various neighbors and doctors of other denominations testified in her defense. One doctor called her "the most intelligent lady I have talked with in many years," and said, "I did not agree with her in sentiment on many things, but I do not call people insane because they differ from me" (*Marital* 42-43). After seven minutes of deliberation, the jury came back with the verdict that Elizabeth Packard was sane, and the judge ordered her release from imprisonment.

After her trial, Elizabeth began to fight for the rights of married women around the country. Before Elizabeth's release, her husband had fled the state with their money, belongings, and children. Eager to see her children, Elizabeth followed her family to their hometown in Massachusetts. Afraid that her husband would have her institutionalized in that state, Elizabeth petitioned the Massachusetts legislature to change the law. She asked that "No person be regarded or treated as an Insane person, or a Monomaniac simply for the *expression of opinions*" (Packard, *Marital* 63). This request clearly invokes the first amendment, which guarantees both freedom of speech and freedom of religion. As a result of her petition, the Massachusetts law was revised so that a woman's husband "must now get ten of her nearest relatives to join him in his request" for institutionalization (*Marital* 66). Thanks to Elizabeth Packard, it became harder for women to be institutionalized merely for expressing their beliefs in the state of Massachusetts.

After her wins in Illinois and Massachusetts, Elizabeth Packard publicized her own sufferings in order to protect the right to freedom of opinion for married women throughout the country. She argued that the laws had to be changed "in order that justice may be done to that class of miserable inmates who are unjustly confined there" (Packard, *Marital* 12). She repeatedly spoke of her case as representative of other married women who had been unjustly institutionalized by their husbands. She aimed her books for an audience of reformers who wanted to improve society, especially those concerned with elevating the status of women. While her goal was to change the law, Elizabeth Packard was aware that she needed to target a wider audience than lawmakers in order to protect women in America from being unjustly incarcerated. As Susan Hubert explains, "Her efforts brought national attention to commitment practices and helped promote legislation to prevent the incarceration of sane individuals and to protect the rights of married women" (38). Unfortunately, there were still many other women in nineteenth-century America who were persecuted for standing up for their rights.

In Packard's book, *The Prisoner's Hidden Life* (1868), she includes the testimony of five other women she met while in the asylum, including Sophia Olsen. Although Sophia was not incarcerated for religious reasons, a poem she wrote during her incarceration focuses on the unjust incarceration of women whose religious beliefs challenge those of mainstream society. "Spare the Creed!" is not included in her own testimony, but is situated within the narrative of Elizabeth Packard, indicating that Olsen wrote the poem with her fellow inmate in mind. The poem is told from the perspective of the conservative Christian who will go to any lengths "To protect our darling creed" (14). To "spare the creed," this zealot will "Force the mother from her home! . . . / Bind her fast with maniacs, where / None will heed her darling prayer" (7-10). These asylum narratives often express the belief that the asylum is a place to bury a woman alive so that her voice is silenced, her protests dismissed as that of a maniac. The narrator calls for the woman who challenges religious doctrine to be bound as well as gagged: "Fetter mothers such as these! / Iron manacles we need / To protect our darling creed" (12-14). Like other asylum texts, this poem points to the violation of a woman's inalienable rights: "What were life, love, liberty, / If our creed imperiled be!" (17-18). Olsen unmistakably echoes the rhetoric of the American Revolution in her protest of religious intolerance. The message of Olsen's poem is clear—the asylum is a place where women who boldly challenge religious creeds are silenced and contained, and the State is complicit in their incarceration:

> Thus State power august hath wrought
> Fetters for too daring thought!
> Souls thus bold, Asylums need,
> To protect our precious creed. (21-24)

Olsen suggests here that women's rights as citizens are denied by the state itself.

While in the asylum, Packard met several other women who had been imprisoned because they did not follow the religious creeds of their husbands. One of these women was Tirzah Shedd. In 1865, Tirzah's husband had imprisoned her in the insane asylum for fourteen weeks because of her belief in spiritualism. Shedd was shocked that the law left her "personal liberty entirely in the hands of my husband, who was fully determined to use this legal power to subject my views to his will and wishes" (132). Refusing to bow to her husband and the law, she boldly stood up for her own inalienable rights: "I should never yield my right to my personal liberty to him or any other power; for so long as he could bring nothing against me but what I regarded as my religion, I claimed the protection of my personal liberty under the flag of religious toleration" (132). Shedd repeatedly employs the rhetoric of natural rights by referencing her "personal liberty." According to Shedd, the superintendent of the asylum told her husband that she was not insane, but he agreed to pronounce her so nevertheless because she would not obey her husband. Like Packard, Shedd was disgusted to discover that women were not afforded the same rights as men: "And yet this is a land of religious freedom! It may be a land of freedom for the *men*, but I am sure it is not for the *married women!*" (132-33). Like other woman's rights advocates of the time, Shedd points out the hypocrisy of those who would deny women the freedom of religion guaranteed in the Bill of Rights.

Shedd and Packard were only two of many women who were institutionalized as insane because their religious beliefs differed from those around them. Many other women in the asylum were imprisoned for spiritualism. One reason spiritualism was probably enticing to women was because it was a religion in which women held positions of authority. However, that authority may have been a source of resentment for some men. According to Shedd, "There were a great many spiritualists there, whom [the doctor] called insane like myself, for this reason alone, seeming to fear them as witnessing against him, unless they carried his diploma of 'hopeless insanity' upon them" (134). Sarah Minard, another woman published by Packard, was imprisoned for nine years for her spiritualist beliefs. Employing the rhetoric of natural rights, she exclaims, "All I want, and sigh for, is *religious freedom*—that I may dare to *do right*, and imperil my personal liberty by so doing!" (131). Minard tells of another sane woman imprisoned for spiritualism "whose case represents a large class of patients I saw there. She is a spirit medium, *but not insane*. . . . She shows no evidence of insanity whatever, in her conduct—it is only her opinions she is imprisoned for" (129). In addition to Sarah Minard, Sophia Olsen met many other spiritualists she liked and respected in the asylum. Calling attention to the government's complicity in suppressing rights it is supposed to protect, Olsen writes sarcastically: "If all Spiritualists must be confined in 'Lunatic Asylums,' we shall soon want Uncle Sam to give us an unlimited quantity of government land upon which to erect them!" (*Mrs. Olsen's* 24). Olsen knows of "many others . . . within the class of those whose peculiar religious beliefs does not at all unfit them from performing all their home duties, were they allowed to do so, in the most praiseworthy and exemplary manner" (*Mrs. Olsen's* 120). She asks "Why is she not fit? Because she believes that spirits from Heaven watch over and guide both herself and her children? Because she believes that our religious beliefs ought to be free and untrammeled?" (*Mrs. Olsen's* 119-20). Fortunately, the superintendent was eventually obliged to let many of these spiritualists free (Shedd 134).

Another woman whose testimony is included in *The Prisoner's Hidden Life* is Caroline Lake, a woman whose husband institutionalized her for religious monomania (140). Although Lake does not comment on her own sanity, she does say "I think there are many married women put there to get rid of them, who are not insane at all" (142). Lake claims that her husband offered the Asylum superintendent five hundred dollars upon admission (140). While her husband asserts that this hefty fee was for curing his wife (143), one must imagine that it would be powerful incentive for the doctor to declare Lake insane and accept her as a patient. Most of Lake's testimony focuses on the lack of rights for inmates, rather than her own circumstances. She writes: "The patients get no course of treatment at that Institution, that I could find, but restraint and imprisonment, the loss of their natural rights, and in some cases, great abuse" (140). One right that Lake especially misses is the right to free speech: "it was a course of severe treatment to me, to put me where my word is not regarded" (140). Lake claims that "It is of no use to appeal to [the doctor] while a patient is there. He seems to act as though patients had no rights which he is bound to respect at all" (141). Moreover, patients are not permitted to speak freely to their friends in the outside world. They are not allowed to communicate with friends unless the communications are positive about their asylum experiences, so they must "utter lies by saying that we are well cared for, or we can have no communication with them whatever" (141). Telling the truth about one's experiences in the asylum meets with punishment and further usurpation of rights. When one patient wrote to the brother of another inmate to tell him that his sister was a sane woman falsely imprisoned, the doctor told this good Samaritan that as punishment her duration at the asylum would be extended (142). Lake's husband employs the same rhetoric when he admits, "I can see no reason why the patients should not be allowed to write freely, and just what they please. Every natural social right should be protected to them" (143)—every right except freedom of religion apparently.

Illinois was not the only state in the union that allowed women to be imprisoned in asylums because of their religious beliefs. Phebe Davis was incarcerated at the New York Asylum at Utica for over two years for challenging the religious creeds of her neighbors in Syracuse. The exact circumstances of her admission are unclear, but Davis was incarcerated because "the pious people call me crazy" (50). She sarcastically explains: "It is now twenty-one years since people found out that I was crazy, and all because I could not fall in with every vulgar belief that was fashionable. I never could be led by everything and everybody, simply because they all told me their arguments were right" (47). Although Davis knew her acquiescence to mainstream beliefs would be easier than her opposition, she speaks her mind because "there are circumstances where 'forbearance ceases to be a virtue'" (49). Instead of repressing her true beliefs, Davis chooses to exercise what she understands as her inalienable rights. She quickly learns, however, that "for all we claim freedom of speech, our mouths are subjected to monarchical government just as much as the dogs are to the muzzle" (51). By exercising her rights to freedoms of speech and religion, Davis is defying her prescribed gender role: "Society compels [women] to make their mouth[s] a sealed book" (51). Importantly, Davis recognizes that society expects her to forfeit her individual rights because she is a woman.

Like Elizabeth Cady Stanton, Davis connects the subjugation of women to the Bible:

> There is one old fact that I would like to have die out, which is, that a woman must not speak a loud word because St. Paul said that they must not. What if he did say so, he was only one man in the world, and that was only his opinion; and who cares for the opinion of one love sick old bachelor, after he has been dead for centuries. I have been imprisoned for over two years simply because I presumed to claim my individual rights. (51)

According to Hoffert, early feminists' "fiercest opposition came from the clergy, who decried the kind of world they envisioned and attacked them from pulpit and podium, arguing that the basis for proscribing the activities of women was to be found in the Bible" (58). Advocates like Lucretia Mott responded to such arguments by claiming that "woman's inferior position was not God's work but the work of men who misinterpreted the Bible and structured the hierarchies of religious institutions to devalue and exclude women" (Hoffert 58).

For opposing misogyny and the religious leaders who endorsed it, Davis was punished with imprisonment in an insane asylum. While this was an attempt to silence a woman who refused to silence herself, Davis refused to fold: "they locked me up when they pleased, but what did I care for that as long as they had no key that would fit my mouth. I knew that I should live through it all, and I told them I should, and that when I got out they would hear from me" (49). And they did. Despite being punished for refusing to conform to societal norms, Davis defiantly continued to assert her rights and make her voice heard. She writes proudly, "I can wear them out, which they cannot me, and I still choose my own position" (49-50). *Two Years and Three Months in the New York Lunatic Asylum at Utica* (1855) was one of the first texts published by a woman incarcerated in an insane asylum, and Davis's steadfast refusal to bow to religious pressure makes it one of the most powerful asylum narratives as well.

While many women were institutionalized for religious reasons, economics motivated the institutionalization of others. Sometimes these two issues were linked. As Kate Lee observes in *A Year at Elgin Insane Asylum* (1902), "One who had large possessions might be thought fanatical or insane if she desired to devote her life entirely to Christian service, and might be put into an asylum in order to get her money" (212). And while her pursuit of freedom of religion was the primary motivation behind Elizabeth Packard's incarceration, money came into play as well. Before sending her to the asylum, Packard's husband suggested that she visit her brother for an extended period of time, but he refused to let her take any money. Elizabeth responded: "Well, husband, if I can't be trusted with ten dollars of my own money under these circumstances, I should not think I was capable of being trusted with two sick children three months away from home, wholly dependent on a poor brother's charities" (*Prisoner's* 1: 35). Apparently asking for money is the last straw for Mr. Packard, as he immediately screams: "You have lost your last chance. You *shall* go into an Asylum!" (*Prisoner's* 1: 35).

Sadly, there were many men who begrudged their wives economic freedom. Alice Russell mentions several in her narrative, *A Plea for the Insane by Friends of the Living Dead* (1898). When one woman decided to gain "independence" by accepting a job as a janitress, her husband immediately had his wife committed to an asylum (Russell 196). When another woman borrowed money to feed her family because her husband was out of work, he quickly had her "committed to the asylum with no friends at hand to interfere" (Russell 196). Evidently it was not unheard of for an unemployed man to put his wife in the asylum for trying to get money to live on. Adriana Brincklé knew one such woman who is in the asylum with her baby: "I knew her well and was certain that she was not insane. Her husband was thriftless, she sued him for support, and he, out of revenge, put her in the asylum" (196-97). Husbands were not always the one to turn the key, though. Kate Lee knew one woman who "was sent to Elgin by a son-in-law who wanted her out of the house, so that he and his family could live in it" (211). Alice Russell knew of another woman who had been wronged out of some property and was trying to regain it when she was incarcerated in the asylum (197).

Perhaps Alice Russell remembered so many stories about women who were institutionalized for standing up for their economic rights because that was the reason she was imprisoned as well. According to Russell, she "refuse[d] to sell her property to suit the caprice of her husband," so he, "acting on the advice of a lawyer," had her committed to an asylum (195). She writes: "Dear reader, just stop a moment and think this is yourself. A sheriff calls in the early morning; you are at your accustomed duties; have had no sickness to prevent you for your usual labors; he reads you a warrant for your arrest; to be examined for insanity. The complainant is your husband" (Russell 192). Alice reportedly had no opportunity to rally her friends for support before she was taken to the asylum (198). Before she knew what was happening, she had "become a public charity" and her husband was in possession of her $20,000 (196). Alice warns her readers "if you will but make even so little investigation into the methods used to commit people, you will with terror admit that you or no one is safe" (194). Sanity cannot save you. Alice's doctor even told her that he knew she was not insane, "but was placed there for other reasons" (198). Now, instead of having economic independence, she is a "slave" in the asylum (193), and her "complaints are compensated by additional abuse" (Russell 194).

Although Alice was worth quite a bit of money, other women were committed for far less. Elizabeth Packard knows of at least one woman who was placed in the asylum for asserting her economic independence. According to Packard, Mrs. Sullivan's husband was a drunk who "showed his regard for his wife in the same manner that Mr. Packard, and many other husbands do, by legally committing her to Dr. McFarland's protection" (*Modern* 171). Evidently this "quick-tempered Irishman" committed his wife to the asylum "because she asserted her inalienable right to a new pair of shoes" (*Modern* 171). Mrs. Simpson's complaints, like those of Alice and the other women at the asylum, do no good, as her words are "listened to as the ravings of a maniac!" (*Modern* 171). Moreover, Packard claims that the superintendent tortures Mrs. Sullivan "for the benevolent purpose of making her willing to return to her husband and yield unanswering obedience to this marital subjection!" (*Modern* 171-72). Packard argues that abused women like Mrs. Sullivan need protection instead of punishment: "But no, the 'lords of creation' must be protected! or oppressed woman will rise and assert her rights, and man then will fail to keep her down" (*Modern* 173). As in her defense of freedom of expression and religion, Packard employs the language of natural rights to defend women's economic independence.

Like Mrs. Sullivan, Adriana Brincklé was committed to the asylum because of economic extravagance. According to Brincklé, her father and uncle had always paid her debts until the summer of 1857, when both of their business investments went bad. She had run up a debt with a merchant that her family could not pay, so the merchant was taking her to court. Like Alice Russell's husband, Brincklé's father sought legal advice about what to do. His good friend, who happened to be on the Supreme Court of Pennsylvania, was Mr. Brincklé's advisor. Rather than face the embarrassment of a trial, the judge advised her father to have Brincklé declared insane and committed to an asylum. Because her father was a physician, he only needed one other signature to have his daughter committed. Brincklé describes the brief examination that sent her to the asylum: "My father asked me a few simple questions and then took his departure. The late Dr. George McClellan, the other examiner, inquired how I was in bodily health. I complained merely of a slight headache, having no idea that the visit was made with an alleged view of determining my mental condition" (191). Her father didn't even accompany her to the asylum. The judge who had been the mastermind behind Brincklé's institutionalization was her escort, as he tried to reconcile her that "insanity was after all the bluntest horn of the dilemma because it preserved family honor" (192). When admitting her, the judge identified her "extravagant tendencies" as the reason for her incarceration to the asylum superintendent and matron (192). Brincklé's father only came to visit her once, a year later, when "He promised me that if I would wait until the troubles caused by my debts had blown over he would have me released. Then he went away. I never saw him again, and he died four years later" (193). Brincklé wasn't released until 1885—twenty-eight years after her admittance—when a change in Pennsylvania law allowed women to appeal their institutionalization. However, upon release Brincklé was destitute, as her inheritance had been used to pay her board at the asylum. If her story sounds too incredible, she assures her readers that it can be verified by the Committee on Lunacy of the Board of Public Charities of Pennsylvania.

While many women were imprisoned in insane asylums for religious and economic reasons, some were admitted for purely domestic reasons. According to Clarissa Lathrop, she knew "a poor widow was incarcerated there who was perfectly sane" (155). A doctor in her village had told the widow to do the washing for his family, but she had refused—as punishment she was sent to the asylum. Kate Lee knew many women were sent to the asylum "for family troubles of various kinds" (211). According to Sophia Olsen, some girls were admitted to the madhouse as punishment for losing their virginity (*Mrs. Olsen's* 117). Alice Russell reportedly heard the superintendent tell one woman, "Your husband don't want you; he told me so; you're no good at home" (199). Caroline Lake writes, "I think there are many married women put there to get rid of them, who are not insane at all" (142). One such woman wrote the poem "Scene in a Private Mad-House" (1842). She begs the jailor to listen to her story, saying "I am not mad, I am not mad! / My tyrant husband forged the tale / which chains me in this dismal cell" (8-10). Tirzah Shedd reportedly knew a sane woman whose husband had admitted her seven times in the same year (136). Sophia Olsen says that sometimes a woman is put in the asylum "[i]f a man becomes tired of living with his wife, and finds affections being alienated from her because she has outlived her beauty and become prematurely old, and her health has decayed in her arduous labors for himself and for their children" (*Mrs. Olsen's* 117). Perhaps that is what happened to her, for her husband sent her to the asylum too, though she doesn't explain why. One night after hearing an inmate lament, "husband may you never know, the doom of sorrow and of woe, you have assigned to me, who once shared your pillow!" the two women "wept in concert, though separated by locks and keys" (*Mrs. Olsen's* 38-39).

Some women in the asylum are victims of domestic abuse. Elizabeth Packard claims that Sophia Olsen came to the asylum willingly when her husband suggested it because *he* was insane and brutally abusing *her* (*Prisoner's* 2: 7). Alice Russell also knows victims of domestic violence. She says that Mrs. Harms and her daughter were starved and beaten by Mr. Harms (201). When he had his wife institutionalized, his daughter ran away from home to be with her mother at the asylum. Although the daughter was able to vouch for her mother's sanity, the mother was not released. Like Sophia Olsen, Mrs. Harms seems to be the dual victim of unjust imprisonment and domestic abuse (Russell 201). Lizzie Cottier is also an asylum victim who has suffered domestic violence. In the preface to *The Right Spirit* (1885), Cottier explains how her husband threatened to separate her from their children if she didn't stop complaining about the abuse. When she covertly handed her children off to some friends, her husband retaliated by admitting her to the asylum (Cottier 6).

Some women's narratives suggest that the asylum is a place where bold women are punished. Women who misbehave are sent to the lower wards, where they are progressively more mistreated. Sophia Olsen is "sent down" after she threatens to tell the superintendent of an attendant's abusive behavior (*Mrs. Olsen's* 45). There, Olsen says, "was exacted the most immediate and uncompromising obedience to rules and requirements which a slave holder would have blushed to inflict upon his human chattels" (*Mrs. Olsen's* 51). When Olsen begs the matron of the lowest wards to lock her in her own cell so that she cannot be brutalized by insane inmates, the matron refuses to help her, saying: "ye ain't crazy, un ye must have been ugly, or yur friends wouldn't put ye into sich a place as this . . . un ye needn't be complainin iny more to me. If they kill ye, 'tis likely ye deserve it" (*Mrs. Olsen's* 68). In retaliation for abuse, one of the women forms a mission to irritate the asylum matron. She secretly destroys all the blankets, the glassware, and the crockery, and disposes of the soap, the brooms, and the silverware (*Mrs. Olsen's* 86). When the woman eventually confesses, she is promptly put in a straitjacket and taken to the lowest ward, never to be seen again.

While Sophia Olsen's story only suggests that women are punished into submission, other narratives are more explicit. Tirzah Shedd writes: "This house seems to me to be more of a place of punishment than a place of cure" (136). Sarah Minard claims: "The great object of the Institution seems to be to subject the patient to the will of the persecutor" (129). Minard writes of the arbitrary and degrading rules of the asylum, like forcing the women to dress in front of everyone in the halls every morning. She believed it was "only an effort to break them down into a state of abject subjection as dependent menials" (127). According to Minard, when patients arrive at the asylum they are immediately put in the bath and "oftentimes are held completely under the water, until almost dead, before they allow them the chance to breathe. . . . This treatment is afterwards used as a threat, ever overhanging them, in case of any resistance to the will or wishes of those who rule over them" (Minard 128). Through threats and violence, the insane asylum trains patients to be submissive.

Always astute and eloquent, Elizabeth Packard portrays the institution as a place where men can send their wives to be tamed as well. Packard argues that many husbands are guilty of "falsely accusing [their wives] of insanity, and once branded by Dr. McFarland's diploma of 'hopelessly insane,' they fondly think they can keep her under their feet" (*Modern* 175). She continues: "Yes, the modern mode of subjugating a married woman is, to send her off to an insane asylum and get her publicly branded as 'hopelessly insane.' Thus, instead of the husband whipping his own wife . . . he sends her off to an insane asylum to get the officials of that institution to whip her for him!" (*Modern* 175). Packard asks sarcastically: "Oh, when this great Woman Subjector, Dr. McFarland, is exposed, where will these men send their wives to get them 'broke in'? Oh! where?" (*Modern* 174).

The scenes described in asylum narratives are often sickening. Not only is the brutal treatment of the inmates horrifying, it is horrifying to think of a sane woman being locked in an asylum among lunatics. Usually, there is some small consolation for the poor victim—she is not alone. As I have attempted to show, there are many more narratives written by women protesting their institutionalization than one would ever imagine. What is even more appalling than the number of these narratives, though, is the number of stories about other women who never wrote a narrative. Each of these authors rattles off tales of other inmates unjustly imprisoned. We owe so much to the women who "felt it was their duty to write not only for themselves but for the women who were locked away and who did not have the means to tell their own stories" (Geller and Harris 5). As Adeline Lunt writes in *Behind Bars* (1871), "it would be incessantly proved that the asylum was supported by a class who *need not be there*. There are two thirds or more on average of such patients in asylums" (256). We must, finally, agree with Elizabeth Cady Stanton to be shocked at the number of "rebellious wives, sisters, and daughters who are thus sacrificed" to the asylum. These women were sacrificed for a number of reasons, but most commonly they were punished for asserting their religious, economic, and domestic rights.

Many of the women unjustly locked in the asylums were not the typical women of nineteenth-century America. Countless were subjected to punishment because they refused to submit to the limitations men and society placed on them. These women were reformers, and they embraced that role. Kate Lee writes, "It is probable that in the course of the world's history a number have been considered insane whom posterity would not regard in that light. Among these are reformers" (212). Always humble, Packard calls herself "a pioneer, just about twenty-five years in advance of my contemporaries,—therefore, I am called crazy, or insane, by those so far in my rear, that they cannot see the reasonableness of the positions and opinions I assume to advocate and defend" (*Exposure* 7). Indeed, twenty-five years may be selling herself short. Phebe Davis observes, "real high souled people are but little appreciated in this world—they are never respected until they have been dead two or three hundred years" (49). Perhaps this is why these narratives lay forgotten somewhere, covered in dust on a library shelf. Perhaps the world still isn't ready to fully respect these high-souled women. Or perhaps America wants to forget its dark past.

Sophia Olsen predicted that "the inhabitants of the Twentieth century . . . will regard this prison with the same feelings as we now do the Spanish Inquisition" (*Mrs. Olsen's* 46). Similarly, Ada Metcalf compares herself to "a slave—in one of those 'Inquisitorial Prisons'" (131). Like the victims of the Spanish Inquisition, many of these women refused to bow down to tyranny. They faced torture rather than relinquish their religious beliefs and their human rights. Metcalf also compares the ostracism of bold women in asylums to the treatment of so-called witches in previous centuries: "The witches are still hung; and the people, unknowingly are aiding and abetting the deed!" (Metcalf 125). Elizabeth Packard agrees: "Much that is now called insanity will be looked upon by future ages, with a feeling similar to what we feel towards those who suffered as witches, in Salem, Massachusetts" (*Modern* 95). Like the victims of the Salem Witch Trials, many of these women refused to conform to society. Instead of being labeled a heretic and burned at the stake, or labeled a witch and sent to the gallows, they were labeled mad and sent to the asylum.

In comparing the unjust institutionalization of women to the Spanish Inquisition and the Salem Witch Trials, the authors of these asylum narratives link the discrimination of women in nineteenth-century America to other forms of discrimination throughout history. Such references serve the same purpose as the references to slavery that highlight the oppression of women in a patriarchal society. Meanwhile, "the language of natural rights and liberal individualism provided [woman's rights advocates] with an ideological framework which helped them to develop their own sense of history and legitimized their right to promote their own self-interests" (Hoffert 71). By protesting gender inequality and employing the same rhetoric as woman's rights advocates, the authors of these asylum narratives identify themselves as part of the woman's rights movement in nineteenth-century America.[3] Thus, these women were not passive victims but active protestors of gender discrimination.[4]

Because these women boldly asserted their own rights and were punished for their assertions with institutionalization, they are an apt illustration of the fight against gender discrimination in nineteenth-century America. Those who opposed the struggle for woman's rights often depicted the advocates of the movement as mentally imbalanced, presumably for no other reason than that they were standing up for themselves and stepping

---

[3] According to Sylvia Hoffert, "Use of this particular set of metaphors testified to membership in the community of woman's rights reformers and the like-mindedness of its participants" (72).

[4] As Hoffert points out, "Personal circumstances determined which aspects of gender discrimination triggered feminist consciousness and brought individual women into the woman's rights movement" (9). Advocates were inspired to join the cause after witnessing gender discrimination in various places, including temperance groups, anti-slavery groups, church groups, the workplace, and the courtroom.

outside of their prescribed gender role. The *New York Herald* described organizers of the first National Woman's Rights Convention held in 1850 as "fugitive lunatics" and supporters of the cause as a "class of wild enthusiasts and visionaries—very sincere, but very mad" (qtd. in Hoffert 97). Indeed, six years later the *Herald* labeled woman's rights conventions "the gatherings of an insane asylum" (qtd. in Hoffert 98).[5] Due to the cultural association between women and mental illness, women in nineteenth-century America who defied societal conventions by standing up for themselves risked being labeled "mad," as these asylum narratives vividly illustrate.

[5] According to Hoffert, such characterizations of woman's rights advocates in the *Herald* was consistent throughout the 1850s (97).

CHAPTER FOUR

"ECCENTRIC AND UNMANAGEABLE": MARY LINCOLN'S LEGACY OF LUNACY

Various women in the nineteenth and early twentieth centuries were institutionalized for unconventional behavior and religious beliefs, but the most famous of these was Mary Lincoln. In 1875 Mary Lincoln's only surviving son Robert had her tried for insanity and placed in an asylum. Soon afterwards, Mary began a campaign to free herself, insisting that she was the sane victim of a heartless son who had her institutionalized for selfish motives. While there is much debate among historians as to whether or not Mary Lincoln was insane, her contemporaries generally agreed that she was. She was a domineering, temperamental, quick-witted woman during a time when society expected women to be silent, submissive, and supportive. Over the years, her unconventional behavior caused many people to question her sanity. While Mary was institutionalized in the spring of 1875, her sanity was questioned long before this. Certain aspects of Mary's life lie at the center of the controversy surrounding her sanity: her domineering personality, her expenditures, her mourning, and her spiritualism. To understand the case of Mary Lincoln, we must consider all of these issues. Such an examination reveals that she was ultimately punished for behaving in ways that society deemed "eccentric and unmanageable" ("Clouded Reason" 20). However, like the authors of asylum narratives, Mary Lincoln protested her diagnosis and her punishment.

Sources spanning from the nineteenth century until the modern day provide conflicting views of Mary Lincoln. One of Abraham Lincoln's first biographers, William Herndon, was the president's former law partner and Mary's enemy. The year after Lincoln's assassination, Herndon embarked on a series of public lectures in which he bad-mouthed Mary. His biography of Lincoln published in 1889 takes the same tone and has had a lasting impact on Mary's legacy. In 1928, Honoré Wilsie Morrow published a biography of Mary Lincoln meant to recuperate the First Lady's tarnished image. Morrow was a novelist who wrote historical fiction, but she spent ten years researching the lives of the Lincolns for a trilogy of fictional books before she wrote the biography. Historian Jean Baker also attempted to restore Mary Lincoln's reputation in her 1989 biography of the First Lady, but these revisionist histories were rejected by historian Michael Burlingame in his 1994 book on the president. Though Burlingame resuscitated the negative image of Mary described by Herndon, more recent biographies published by Stephen Berry (2007) and Catherine Clinton (2009) have adopted a more neutral tone, though Clinton's ultimately offers a sympathetic view of the First Lady.

Some of Mary's qualities that draw the admiration of modern historians like Baker and Clinton raised eyebrows in her own time. She was devoted to her studies, staying in school much longer than most girls. Moreover, Mary had an unwomanly love of politics and did not hesitate to have an intellectual debate with the men she met, a woman too intellectual and not submissive enough to suit many in Victorian society. She devoted herself to her husband's career. By all accounts, Lincoln would not have ended up in the White House if not for the persistent encouragement of his wife. Even her detractors acknowledged as much. "There is no doubt," William Herndon writes, "that much of Lincoln's success was in a measure attributable to her" (Herndon and Weik 186). Burlingame admits that "Lincoln's ambition was not all-consuming and probably would have not led him to aspire to the presidency had his wife not goaded him on" (254). A more generous commentator agrees: "I am firmly convinced that without Mary Todd Lincoln, the world never would have known Abraham Lincoln, for he never would have reached the White House without her" (Morrow 13). As Morrow explains: "Mary gave the force of her personality to moving Lincoln forward in his career" (82). Morrow claims that Mary spent time "educating him" on proper dress and manners (78). In addition to lessons in manners, Mary made suggestions about his speeches and summarized books that he lacked time to read (Morrow 84).

Mary Lincoln was her husband's chief advisor for most of their marriage. However, after Lincoln's election to the presidency her ability to influence his political decisions dropped dramatically. As Catherine Clinton explains, "Mrs. Lincoln was increasingly supplanted as her husband's domestic adviser and sounding board, elbowed aside by both his official Cabinet and a retinue of young, ambitious men on staff" (157). Wives were supposed to be silent and submissive, and Lincoln's new advisors were shocked and appalled when Mary tried to weigh in on her husband's decisions (Baker 180). These men "resented her unseemly usurpation of their authority" and considered her political interests inappropriate for a woman (Baker 134-35). Although her advice had helped Lincoln rise to the White House, "her unconventional attachment to politics was viewed as a threat, not an asset, by many of Lincoln's supporters and, indeed, the wider world" (Clinton 118). A woman whose husband had always valued her opinions was now labeled "a meddling deviant" (Baker 135). However, Mary Lincoln did not relinquish her advisory role willingly. Indeed, "she desperately clung to her role as consigliere" and resented those who "failed to recognize her primary and vital role as her husband's sounding board" (Clinton 116). Her loss of control was undoubtedly difficult for Mary to accept and probably contributed to her scandalous behavior while in the White House.

Mary's contemporaries were appalled by the money she spent decorating the White House. When the Lincolns moved in, the White House was horribly run-down. Walls and floors were stained with tobacco juice, rugs were bare, and pieces were cut out of the curtains (Morrow 91; Clinton 130). Visitors were shocked that the residence of the President of the United States "resembled a second-rate hotel" (Clinton 130). Mary decided to transform "the tattered and decaying symbol of the nation" (Clinton 136). By doing so, she aimed to impress the world and prove herself as First Lady (Clinton 154). Her plan backfired. Although Congress had allowed the Lincolns $20,000 to redecorate, Mary went over budget (Baker 188). She was not the first person to do so, but Mary was already a target for criticism (Baker 188). Her expenditures prompted condemnation that was "relentless and unreasonable" (Clinton 151). Baker defends Mary Lincoln's purchases, suggesting that her critics did not understand Mary's "purpose of representing her country through high standards of elegance and fashion" (195). Clinton points out that $20,000 was "inadequate to the task" and "paltry compared to other Congressional appropriations for District expenditures at the time" (135). Moreover, it was significantly less than the $125,000 Congress granted Andrew Johnson's family four years later (Clinton 135).

Mary also faced criticism for the money she spent on clothes. To be fair, her expenditures in this department are somewhat understandable as well. Washington was a town of "rigid social hierarchy and intense snobbery," and the established elite "were open in their contempt toward the Lincolns" (Clinton 124). As First Lady, Mary had to appear at a "marathon of exhausting, emotionally draining ceremonies where every aspect of her appearance was critically examined" (Clinton 127). Before the Lincolns even arrived in Washington, Mary was already being criticized for her quaint, Western attire. To remedy the situation, Mary went shopping. Again, her plan backfired. Instead of being praised for her style, Mary was condemned for being a spendthrift. However, this criticism did not prevent Mary from repeating her mistakes. She shopped often and extravagantly. Baker admits Mary spent too much on clothes but suggests she did it to comfort herself when upset. Berry agrees: "For Mary, shopping also satisfied deeper psychological needs. She derived a strange comfort from material possessions" (Berry 55). Mary's contemporaries were not as understanding. When the Lincolns' son Willie died in 1862, the public interpreted it as punishment for Mary's vanity (Baker 215).

Mary Lincoln's responses to the tragedies in her life also garnered harsh criticism from her peers. In the nineteenth century, "Good Christian women knew better than to mourn excessively; visible emotion only displayed their lack of faith" (Baker 211). A woman should bear her losses stoically, proving that she "accepted God's plan" (Berry 186). Mary did not do this. When Willie died, "Mrs. Lincoln's grief was volcanic, as she gave into hysteria and convulsions" (Clinton 167). At one point, Abraham Lincoln allegedly threatened to send her to "that large white building on the hill yonder" that was an insane asylum (qtd. in Neely and McMurtry 3). Mary's grief over Willie's death prevented her from nursing their son Tad, who was seriously ill from the same sickness that had killed his brother (Wheeler 38). Mary stayed in bed for three weeks. After she got out of bed, she continued to avoid people throughout the spring. That summer, the people of D.C. were enraged when Mary cancelled the concert series on the White House grounds because she was in mourning (Baker 216). To her contemporaries, Mary was "a diva of grief whose histrionic performances seemed an unwelcome encore to a life of indulgence and aggrandizement" (Berry 186).

When her husband was shot by an assassin just three years later, Mary was again overcome with grief. Indeed, according to Catherine Clinton "Her grief was so extreme that doctors agreed to withhold the information that there was no expectation of Lincoln's recovery" (2). Nevertheless, Mary could not ignore the obvious. She began to sob hysterically and was eventually banished from the room after she collapsed in a faint. Secretary of War Edwin Stanton reportedly ordered: "Take that woman from the room and do not let her in again" (Clinton 3) (see Fig. 4-1). Not being allowed to attend her husband as he was dying undoubtedly contributed to her grief, as did witnessing the attack at Ford's Theatre. A month later, Mary wrote: "I do not have the least desire to live. . . . God only knows the agony of this crushed heart" (qtd. in Clinton 255). Mary wore widow's weeds for the rest of her life and never recovered from this tragedy. Her only consolation was Tad, as Robert "had neither the temperament nor the inclination to substitute as his mother's comfort" (Clinton 258).

Following Abraham Lincoln's assassination, public criticism of Mary only became more vicious. She was forced to deal with the $25,000 debt she had accrued through shopping. Unsympathetic creditors threatened to sue and demanded repayment. David Davis, the manager of the Lincoln estate, was slow in distributing the inheritance and failed to tell Mary that her share would be one third of $85,000. Desperate, "Mary decided to direct appeals toward some of the rich and powerful men who had grown fat off their appointments by President Lincoln—contacting them, reminding them of their indebtedness, looking for financial handouts" (Clinton 259). Perhaps she would have been more successful if Davis had not told everyone "that [her] means were very ample, and no assistance was required to enable [her] to live *very* comfortably" (Baker 265).

As a last resort, Mary decided to sell some of her clothes to pay off her debts. Before the sale, however, the pawnbroker convinced Mary to write to the men who had made their fortunes off of wartime contracts, suggesting that they owed a debt to the Lincoln family that should be paid. When the letters did not produce the hoped for cash, the pawnbroker put Mrs. Lincoln's wardrobe on public display and published the letters he had persuaded her to write. As Clinton explains, "[n]othing before had ever elicited such a torrent of ridicule" (273). The sale of her clothes became a humiliating exhibition. Moreover, "[t]he public spectacle of Mrs. Lincoln's complaints in print was a terrible breach of Victorian conduct. It was acceptable for men to fight her battles for her, but she was expected to refrain from making any protest, mute on the sidelines" (Clinton 274). Instead of making money, the sale actually cost Mary her money and her reputation. When she received part of her inheritance in the months after the fiasco, Mary fled to Europe in shame with Tad.

The "Old Clothes Scandal" made her son Robert embarrassed and angry. He began excusing his mother by telling people she was insane. According to Jean Baker, "this defense of her behavior was calculated more for the protection of his own respectability than his mother's well-being" (278). While Robert was spared from the humiliation his mother attracted for a few years, she returned to America in 1871. Soon afterwards, her only other living son, Tad, died. Tad had been Mary's sole consolation after the death of her husband. As a result of his passing, she went into another depression. Rather than consoling his bereaved mother, Robert tried to stay as far away from her as possible.

In addition to her excessive mourning, Mary drew attention to herself by practicing spiritualism. After Willie's death, Mary Lincoln began attending séances, even holding several at the White House. Mary believed that the spirit mediums helped her to communicate with her departed sons. During and after the Civil War, many people sought comfort by trying to contact dead loved ones. By 1862, six million Americans subscribed to spiritualism (Clinton 186). Nevertheless, the practice attracted criticism from non-believers. Indeed, some thought belief in the supernatural was a sign of insanity, and many men believed it was sufficient cause to institutionalize their wives and mothers. Abraham Lincoln was not one of these men. He humored his wife, hoping it would give her comfort.[1] His son Robert was not as understanding. Her consultations with spirit mediums after Tad's death was one of the primary reasons Robert believed her to be insane.

In 1875 Robert had his mother tried for insanity. Soon after her incarceration, Mary began insisting that she was sane and that her son had her committed for selfish motives. Thus began the controversy surrounding Mary Lincoln's insanity case. There have been various publications on the subject, and these generally fall into one of two categories: those that accept Robert's side of the story, and those that accept Mary's side of the story. Robert's defenders argue that Mary was, indeed, insane and that Robert had her institutionalized in order to safeguard her own well-being. Mary's defenders portray Robert as a conniving villain who schemed to put his mother behind bars so that he could assume control of her finances and climb the political ladder without the scandalous figure of his mother blocking his ascent.[2] These two polarized views of Mary Lincoln's insanity case generally make it difficult for readers to come to any firm conclusions on the matter. However, an examination of letters, newspaper articles, editorials, interviews, diary entries, legal documents, and patient progress reports from the asylum where Mary was treated[3]—in addition to important contextual information, such as a thorough knowledge of spiritualism—can help us to uncover Mary's mental state and the circumstances surrounding her commitment.

The fact that Mary Lincoln was afforded a trial at all is owing to the efforts of Elizabeth Packard. Because of Packard, a bill was passed in

[1] Most people initially explored Spiritualism because they wished to communicate with a dead loved one (Braude 5). Spiritualist followers were largely seeking comfort, especially through assistance in contacting friends and relatives who had passed away (McGarry 21). Mediums provided that link to the afterlife, delivering messages from the dead who had not departed after all. Mourners found particular consolation in the messages they received from dead loved ones, who were still concerned with the happiness and welfare of the living (Braude 52).

[2] Robert's defenders are either historians like Mark Neely and Gerald McMurtry (1986) who specialize in Abraham Lincoln or historians like Jason Emerson (2007), who specializes in Robert Lincoln. Mary's defenders tend to be either feminist historians like Jean Baker (1986) and Catherine Clinton (2009) or people writing ficitionalized accounts of the trial.

[3] Fortunately, these primary sources have recently been collected and published by Jason Emerson in *Mary Lincoln's Insanity Case: A Documentary History* (2012).

Illinois in 1867 requiring a jury trial for anyone committed to an insane asylum (Neely and McMurtry 21). Alienists of the period thought jury trials were absurd; the very idea was an insult to their expertise and a threat to them. At the time of Mary Lincoln's commitment, jury trials were only required for the commitment of the insane in three states: Illinois, Indiana, and Kentucky (Neely and McMurtry 22). Thus, "Robert was forced to comply with the country's—perhaps the world's—strictest legal standards for the commitment of the insane" (Neely and McMurtry 21). However, these strict legal standards did not ensure that Mary Lincoln was given a fair trial.

During her trial, no mention was made of Mary's spiritualist beliefs. However, this is probably because Robert and his Chicago legal team were careful to avoid the subject of religious toleration after Elizabeth Packard's crusade had changed Illinois laws a few years prior. An examination of Robert's personal papers reveals that Mary's spiritualism was, indeed, one of the primary reasons he believed his mother to be insane. Since her son Willie's death in 1862, Mary had visited mediums and attended séances. She revived her spiritualist activities after the death of her son Tad in 1871. Like many Victorian men, Robert found his mother's belief in spirit communications to be insane and was appalled by the money she spent on mediums.

The other major factor that led Robert and many of his contemporaries to deduce that Mary Lincoln was insane was her shopping habit. The nation had considered Mary to be a spendthrift since her early days in the White House, when she went over budget to redecorate during wartime and spent ungodly amounts on her wardrobe. Unlike her spiritualism, Mary's shopping habits featured prominently in her trial, where Robert paid a long line of merchants to testify to her extravagant purchases and even more hotel workers to testify to how she stashed packages in a closet never to be opened again.

In addition to paying merchants and hotel workers to testify to his mother's shopping habits, Robert also paid six doctors to certify her as insane *without examining her* based on his descriptions of her behavior. Mary Lincoln received no defense from Isaac Arnold, the lawyer that Robert and his legal team had engaged for her. Arnold actually "doubted the propriety of his defending her" (Swett 48)," but Leonard Swett—Robert's head lawyer—told him "you will put into her head, that she can get some mischievous lawyer to make us trouble; go and defend her and do your duty" (Swett 48). If Arnold had actually wanted to summon witnesses and mount a defense for Mary Lincoln, his ability to do so would have been hampered by the fact that the trial was sprung on her at literally the last minute, when

Swett arrived at her hotel room to escort her to court. According to Neely and McMurtry, "Failure to give notice in such cases was a serious offense, and the Illinois Supreme Court had made a ringing pronouncement on the question in 1854" (23). Justice John D. Caton wrote:

> every principle of justice and right requires that [the accused insane] should have notice and be allowed to make manifest his sanity, and to refute or explain the evidence tending to prove the reverse. . . . The idea is too monstrous to be tolerated for a moment, that the legislature ever intended to establish a rule by which secret proceedings might be instituted against any member of the community, by any party who might be interested, to shut him up in a madhouse, by which he might be divested of his property and his liberty, without an opportunity for a struggle on his part. Should such a principle be sustained, the most sane man in the State is liable to be surprised at any moment, by finding himself bereft of his property, and on his way to a lunatic asylum.
> (qtd. in Neely and McMurtry 24)

The lack of notice not only meant that Mary did not have time to mount a defense, it also ensured that Mary was denied the right of participating in the jury selection (Rhodes and Jauchius 15). While these circumstances indicate that Mary Lincoln did not have a fair chance to defend herself, they do not mean that she was sane. Indeed, her sanity is still a question of debate.

Scholars have offered various interpretations of both Mary's and Robert's actions. Always Mary's defender, Jean Baker suggests that Robert committed Mary out of greed. According to Baker, Robert complained that the mediums would eat up his inheritance (323). With her institutionalization, Robert gained control of her finances. Clinton provides a muddled interpretation of the issue. She repeatedly implies that the deaths of her loved ones, financial concerns, and public harassment caused Mary Lincoln to become unhinged. In keeping with this interpretation, Clinton claims that Robert "could see she was in full-blown delusional mode" when he had her committed (Clinton 299). However, Clinton admits that "Mary Lincoln was not given a fair opportunity to oppose her own legal kidnapping" (Clinton 303). Moreover, she points to indications that Robert was just trying to get his mother out of the way: "His promising career in politics was compromised by his mother's erratic behavior. Certainly such considerations must have had an impact on her son's decision" (Clinton 305). To further cloud the issue, Clinton claims that the letters she wrote after the trials "demonstrate Mary Lincoln's steel-trap grasp of the details of her situation," and that "her faculties appear razor-sharp" (323). Clearly there are various interpretations of Mary's mental state and Robert's motives, even within the same book.

Although Robert is portrayed as a "mustache-twirling villain" by some historians who claim Mary was unjustly incarcerated (Emerson xii), others suggest that Robert's motives were pure. According to Neely and McMurtry, Robert Lincoln's political career was limited by "his own detestation of political life, a loathing that Robert himself once described as 'almost morbid'" (78). Therefore, it seems unlikely that Robert would have had his mother committed just so she wouldn't stand in the way of his political ambitions. Documentary evidence also invalidates the suggestion that Robert had her committed because he wanted her money to himself. In a letter consulting David Davis about what to do with his mother's money, Robert suggested that they have "a competent person make an estimate on the annuity principle of what monthly sum can be paid her during her life so as to leave nothing at her death and . . . to pay such sum to her monthly" (154). This seems to prove that his interest in his mother's money was not for self-gain. Moreover, Robert declared in a letter to Ninian Edwards: "I do not desire that any interest of mine or my children in the ultimate disposition of her property should be covenanted and the only object I wish attained by any plan is her own protection" (163). He only acted as his mother's conservator because others refused the office, and as her conservator he actually increased her estate without fee (Neely and McMurtry 142).

While the evidence suggests that Robert did not have his mother committed for his own monetary gain, he did have her committed largely for monetary reasons. In his letters to friends and family, Robert Lincoln repeatedly worries that his mother's excessive expenditures would leave her nothing to live on. However, these letters also reveal another reason that Robert Lincoln committed his mother: embarrassment. Explaining his reasons for institutionalizing his mother, Robert wrote in a letter to Henry Blow: "If my mother were not in such a situation in life that her insane vagaries make national scandals, there might be no harm in letting her do as she chooses" (100). Likewise, when his aunt Elizabeth wrote to Robert expressing her opinion that Mary shouldn't be in an asylum, he replied: "If you have in your mind any plan by which my mother can be placed under care and under some control which might prevent her from making herself talked of by everybody, I hope you will write it to me" (104). Such comments make clear that preventing his mother from causing more embarrassment was a major factor in Robert's decision to institutionalize her.

Robert's primary motives for committing his mother seem to be that he wanted to prevent her from spending all of her money and from creating more scandals. While her shopping habit and her spiritualist beliefs—and whatever embarrassment these things caused—do not seem like adequate reasons to have her committed to the modern reader, Mary Lincoln did exhibit other more worrying symptoms of psychological distress at the time of her commitment, and many of these symptoms were discussed at her trial as well. Unfortunately, the transcript of the trial has disappeared.[4] However, newspaper coverage of the trial still exists. Of course, these sources are problematic because we do not hear Mary's side of the story. As in the trial, Mary does not here have the opportunity to refute her son's claims or explain her own actions in another light. It is important to keep this under consideration when reading about the alleged symptoms of madness reported by others.

One of the doctors who testified at her trial was Dr. Willis Danforth. Danforth testified that he had treated Mrs. Lincoln in November of 1873 "for fever and nervous derangement of the head" ("Clouded Reason" 17).[5] At that time Mary allegedly told Danforth that an Indian spirit "was pulling wires out of her eyes" ("Clouded Reason" 17). When Danforth treated her for "debility of the nervous system" in September of 1874, Mary told him that "she was going to die within a few days, and that she had been admonished to that effect by her [dead] husband. She imagined that she heard raps on a table conveying the time of her death, and would sit and ask questions and repeat the supposed answer the table would give" ("Clouded Reason" 17). When Danforth visited Mary the week prior to the trial, "her former hallucinations appeared to have passed away" ("Clouded Reason" 17).

---

[4] Rhodes and Jauchius have attributed the disappearance of the trial transcripts to Robert Lincoln's nefarious interference. Robert probably did play a role in their disappearance, though not for any nefarious reasons. Robert destroyed many letters his mother wrote in 1875-1876, the years when she exhibited the most severe symptoms of psychological distress (Neely and McMurtry 144). Moreover, he wrote to Elizabeth Edwards, "I would be ashamed to put on paper an account of many of her insane acts—and I allowed to be introduced into evidence only so much as was necessary to establish the case" (Lincoln 103). After the trial, Robert evidently wanted to destroy that evidence as well, as it was a cause for embarrassment to him and a stain on his family's legacy.

[5] Various Chicago newspapers covered the trial—not because it had been publicized beforehand, but because reporters from the major local newspapers were waiting at the Cook County courthouse in the hopes of coming across an interesting story. Emerson has collected accounts of the trial from six different papers in *Mary Lincoln's Insanity Case.* I refer to the account of the trial published in the *Chicago Tribune* because it seems the most straightforward and comprehensive.

Several other doctors also testified at the trial. Dr. Davis, who had treated her years ago, testified that "he saw nothing in her to indicate unsoundness of mind. She was eccentric and suffered from nervousness" ("Clouded Reason" 20). Though a couple of the doctors had treated Mrs. Lincoln in years past, others had never met her and based their opinion of her mental state on the observations of others. Dr. Johnson testified that the evidence indicated that she was deranged, and Dr. Smith testified that the lack of motives for her strange actions indicated that "her mind was not sound" ("Clouded Reason" 21).

Robert Lincoln paid several hotel employees to testify against his mother. Samuel Turner, the manager of the Chicago hotel Mrs. Lincoln was staying at, testified that Mrs. Lincoln appeared in his office on the day of April 1st saying that there was "a strange man in the corridor" and "she was afraid to be left alone" ("Clouded Reason" 17). Turner thought "her appearance was wild," and he "believed her deranged" ("Clouded Reason" 18). The hotel housekeeper, Mrs. Allen, testified that Mrs. Lincoln "seemed to suffer from nervous excitement," that she had witnessed Mrs. Lincoln pace the room at night, and that she had witnessed Mrs. Lincoln mix several of her medicines together ("Clouded Reason" 18). Another hotel employee testified that Mrs. Lincoln believed people were speaking to her through the walls, and that she was afraid the city would burn down ("Clouded Reason" 18). Mrs. Lincoln had expressed her fear that the city would burn down, as well as her fear of being molested by a strange man who was following her, to various people.

Robert testified that his mother had sent a telegram from Florida in March of 1875 to his law partner, expressing concern that Robert was ill. Robert responded to his mother's telegram, telling her he was fine and that she should remain in Florida. Despite this, Mrs. Lincoln came to Illinois to reassure herself that Robert was not dying. Robert considered this unfounded belief in his illness as evidence of her insanity. He, therefore, hired a man to follow and watch her. Robert also thought his mother was insane because she feared Chicago would burn down, she thought someone had tried to poison her on the train, she claimed that a wandering Jew had taken her pocketbook, and she thought that someone was speaking to her through the walls ("Clouded Reason" 19). Robert testified that his mother "had been of unsound mind since the death of her husband, and had been irresponsible for the last ten years. He regarded her as eccentric and unmanageable" ("Clouded Reason" 20).

Thus, Mary Lincoln was sent to the asylum because she was "eccentric and unmanageable." Yet, even if one is inclined to dismiss her spiritualism and shopping habit, the other symptoms described at this trial make Mary Lincoln seem mentally disturbed. However, we must remember that she had no opportunity to defend herself or accumulate witnesses of her own. The witnesses who appeared were paid by Robert, and they described her behavior without providing any context or suggesting any reasons for that behavior. Mary evidently disagreed with much of this testimony, as reported by a reporter from the *Chicago Times*: "Occasionally as a witness was giving his testimony, she would turn her head toward her counsel, and seem to protest against the assertions being made, and several times her voice was heard in low but vehement denunciation of the proceedings" ("Sad Revelation" 25-26). Unfortunately, we may never know what her objections to the testimony were.

While it is impossible to know what Mary Lincoln's response to the testimony would have been, placing her symptoms in the context of her circumstances may help us to understand and—to some extent—excuse them. Various witnesses testified that Mrs. Lincoln thought she was being followed by a strange man and was afraid that he was going to molest her. While this testimony was framed in such a way as to suggest that Mrs. Lincoln was delusional, in fact Mary Lincoln *was* being followed by a strange man. Robert himself testified that, unbeknownst to his mother, he had hired a Pinkerton guard to follow her around Chicago. And while her fear that Chicago was going to burn down was the other major phobia that people testified to in Mary Lincoln's trial, this phobia is also understandable when placed in context. Just four years prior to the trial was the Great Chicago Fire, when hundreds had died and much of the city was destroyed in a fire that raged for three days (see Fig. 4-2).

Aside from these phobias, witnesses testified that Mary exhibited other delusional symptoms. However, the necessary context for understanding these symptoms was intentionally omitted. Robert and his legal team were careful to avoid the subject of spiritualism at trial due to Elizabeth Packard's recent crusade for religious toleration. While witnesses avoided the mention of spiritualism, they did not refrain from mentioning her spiritualist beliefs. When taken out of this context, however, these beliefs undoubtedly make Mary appear delusional.

Mary's interaction with mediums could actually explain most of her symptoms. Several witnesses reported that Mary believed people were communicating with her through raps on the walls and furniture. While this belief seems like a symptom of a disturbed mind, it was a commonly held belief of spiritualists. Mediums often claimed that the dead communicated to them through a spiritual telegraph, tapping on walls and furniture as they called out the letters of the alphabet.[6] Thus, when Mary told witnesses that people communicated to her this way, she may have meant spirits. She was undoubtedly encouraged in such beliefs by the mediums who visited her. Robert's lawyer, Leonard Swett, wrote that "Pinkerton's man reported that she was being visited in her room by persons regarded by us as suspicious" (Swett 45). At least one mysterious visitor was "presumed to be a prominent Spiritualist" ("Mrs. Lincoln: A Visit" 88). Furthermore, spirit mediums sometimes claimed they could predict the future through the spirits who spoke to them, and that they channeled spirits of the dead while in a trance. If a medium visiting Mary was claiming to channel President Lincoln, this may explain why Mary thought her husband had revealed the day that she would die. This would not be the first time that Mary was taken in by someone claiming to channel a dead loved one. A few years prior to the trial Mary visited the studio of William Mumler, a spiritual photographer who took the infamous picture of Mary with the ghost of her husband watching over her (see Fig. 4-3).[7] Mary's consultations with mediums may also explain why she suddenly became persuaded that her son Robert was dying,

[6] Spiritualism was born on March 31, 1848, in upstate New York, when nighttime noises disturbed the tranquility of the Fox farm. When Mrs. Fox confronted her adolescent daughters—Maggie and Kate—the girls pled innocence, insisting that the loud rappings that echoed through the house were made by a spirit that responded to their questions. Mrs. Fox summoned the neighbors as witnesses to the spirit communications, and the movement spread from there. As news about the supernatural occurrences in the Fox household reached across the country and over the Atlantic, others—especially young girls—quickly discovered that they too had the special ability to communicate with the spirits of the dead. Forty years after Maggie and Kate Fox inadvertently spawned the spiritualist movement, Maggie confessed before a packed crowd in New York that she and Kate had produced the noises by cracking their toe joints upon the bed. They had only meant to tease their superstitious mother.

[7] Mumler claimed that he had the unique ability to photograph the spirits that lingered over their loved ones, and he charged an exorbitant amount for his photographs. Evidently Mary Lincoln did not want to attract attention when she went to Mumler's studio, for she went incognito as Mrs. Lindall. However, her true identity was quickly discovered. When she returned to the studio to retrieve her portrait, she refrained from identifying the spirit, probably in an attempt to retain her privacy. In response, Mrs. Mumler suddenly seemed to become possessed by the spirit of little Tad Lincoln, saying "Mother, if you cannot recognize father, show the picture to Robert; he will recognize it" (qtd. in Cox 114). Mrs. Lincoln responded by bursting into tears. Mumler was eventually tried for fraud, though he was acquitted, in part thanks to the testimony of a spiritualist judge who leant him credibility (Cox 119).

as this could have been another prediction made by a medium claiming to be in contact with the spirit world.

Even the claim that an Indian spirit was pulling wires in her head can be explained in the context of spiritualism. Many mediums, including at least two that Mary Lincoln consulted, claimed that the spirits who possessed them were Indians. In her Washington years, Mary had attended séances presided over by Nettie Colburn Maynard, whose spirit guide was reportedly an Indian maiden named Little Pinkie (Neely and McMurtry 81). Later Mary spent several months amongst a spiritualist community in St. Charles, Illinois, where she daily visited a medium named Mrs. Howard who claimed to be controlled by an Indian doctor ("Mrs. Lincoln: She is Recovering" 121-22). Perhaps these mediums pretended to summon their Indian spirit guides to help heal Mary's headaches. Summoning spirit guides to heal the ill was also a common practice of mediums. While her belief in such mediums may indicate that Mary Lincoln was gullible, it does not indicate that she was insane.[8] Taken out of context in the trial, however, her spiritualist beliefs would certainly appear like symptoms of insanity.

Of course, the lawyer Robert hired for Mary did not call her to the stand to explain her behavior. As a result of the one-sided trial, Mary was committed to a private asylum. The trial was yet another traumatic experience for Mary, and it took its toll. The night of the trial, she went to three different drug stores trying to obtain a deadly combination of laudanum and camphor but was thwarted in her suicide attempt by a savvy pharmacist (Neely and McMurtry 34-35). The next morning, she was committed to a private asylum in Batavia, Illinois that served as a home for a "select class of lady patients of quiet unexceptional habits" who suffered from nervous and mental illnesses (qtd. in Emerson, *Madness* 71). According to a *Chicago Post and Mail* correspondent, "Many of the patients at this place ARE NOT MAD. They are upon what Robert Dale Owen calls debatable land" ("Mrs. Lincoln: A Visit" 89). Since Owen was a famous spiritualist who wrote two books on the subject—one of which was entitled *Debatable Land*—the correspondent seems to be insinuating that many of the asylum patients at Batavia are spiritualists.[9] The patients in Batavia received the "moral treatment" for insanity: "rest, diet, baths, fresh air, occupation, diversion, change of scene, no more medicine than . . . absolutely necessary, and the least restraint possible" (qtd. in Emerson,

[8] As Molly McGarry points out, spiritualism "was popularized in an era when anything seemed possible, when speaking to the dead may have seemed no less strange than communicating across cables or capturing the living on film" (20).

[9] Owen is best remembered as a nineteenth-century social reformer and co-founder of the utopian community of New Harmony, Indiana.

Madness 71). In keeping with the "moral treatment," the asylum at Batavia was located in an idyllic rural setting on the banks of the Fox River and surrounded by manicured lawns, flower gardens, and greenhouses. Not only were there hammocks and lawn chairs for patients to enjoy the outdoors, there were carriages and sleighs available as well (Emerson, *Madness* 71).

Mary remained a patient in the asylum for nearly four months. Her daily progress reports mention no delusions, only bouts of melancholy, restlessness, and depression. In July Mary decided to take an active role in protesting her confinement. She wrote to Judge James Bradwell asking him to visit her at the asylum with his wife. With the help of the Bradwells, Mary was eventually released. Myra Bradwell visited Mary Lincoln repeatedly in the asylum and joined the campaign to free her friend, writing to Mary's sister Elizabeth, Robert, and the newspapers that she "saw not one symptom of insanity" in Mary (109). Both Robert and Dr. Patterson—the physician overseeing Mary at the asylum—were irritated by the interference of the meddlesome Bradwells. Dr. Patterson wrote to Myra Bradwell asking her to "secure [Robert Lincoln's] approval" before visiting Mrs. Lincoln again and to refrain from "conveying any letters that Mrs. Lincoln may write" (107). Clearly Dr. Patterson and Robert Lincoln wanted to thwart the campaign to free Mary. They only agreed to release Mary to her sister's care when Judge James Bradwell wrote to Dr. Patterson: "I, as her legal advisor and friend, will see if a habeas corpus cannot open the door of Mrs. Lincoln's prison house" (119). Judge Bradwell also forced Robert's hand by falsely telling the papers on August 23rd that Dr. Patterson had signed a certificate of release and that Robert Lincoln was going to withdraw her from the asylum later in the week ("Mrs. Lincoln: Startling Interview" 125).

After her release from the asylum, Mary returned to Springfield to stay with her sister Elizabeth Edwards. In September, Elizabeth wrote a letter to Robert saying that everyone in Springfield found Mary "looking . . . well, and in every respect acting in the most agreeable manner" (145). By November, Elizabeth told Robert that she had "no hesitation, in pronouncing her sane, and far more reasonable, and gentle, than in former years" (147). When Elizabeth's husband Ninian Edwards wrote to Robert that same month, he noted an exception to Mary's reasonableness: "Except on the subject of the restoration of her bonds and purchases, she is as rational as I ever knew her" (155). When he wrote to Robert the following January, Ninian noted that Mary's shopping habit was back in full-force: "She spends nearly ½ of every day with dressmakers and in the stores" (167). She was a hoarder, buying and hiding her purchases from others. A second trial to determine Mary's competency was held a year after the first, and Robert and his legal team agreed not to oppose her petition to be declared competent—not because they thought she was competent, but because keeping Mary Lincoln confined seemed like it would cause more trouble and scandal than letting her free. Though Ninian and Elizabeth Edwards had advocated for Mary's release, two days after her trial in June of 1876, Ninian told Robert: "[I] regret very much that the verdict stated that she was 'restored to her reason.' . . . A person may be insane and yet capable of taking care of his property" (185). Though Mary continued to entertain her shopping habit, she managed to live for several more years on her own without causing any spectacles or finding herself destitute.

Though Mary Lincoln was ultimately declared competent and released, her sanity is still a matter of debate. The testimony from the first trial portrays Mary Lincoln as someone whose mind is deeply disturbed. However, Mary was not allowed to respond to this testimony. If she had taken the stand in her own defense, she may have been able to satisfactorily explain her actions by providing the necessary context for them. However, it is also possible that Mary Lincoln was suffering from a mental illness. Indeed, the various traumas she suffered would be explanation enough for such distress. As Elizabeth Edwards told Myra Bradwell after the first trial, "The sorrows that befell her in such rapid succession and *the one*, so tragic, was enough to shatter the nerves, and infuse the intellect of the bravest mind and heart" (98). However, though Elizabeth and her husband at times conceded that Mary might be psychologically disturbed, they did not believe she belonged in an asylum.

Long before the 1875 trial that led to her institutionalization, Mary was accused by many of her contemporaries of being insane. To Mary's enemies, interfering in politics, shopping too much, accruing debs, begging for money, mourning too excessively, and consulting spiritualists were all signs of insanity. Moreover, Jean Baker suggests that Mary was persecuted because she "trampled the canons of womanhood" (325). To some extent this is true. Mary "was a woman of intense intellect and passion who stepped outside the boundaries her times prescribed and suffered for it" (Clinton 336). She was too opinionated and not submissive enough to suit Victorian society. While Mary Lincoln's purportedly unwomanly behavior caused some to label her "mad" well before the trial that sent her to an asylum, the primary reasons for her commitment were her shopping, her spiritualism, and the embarrassment she caused her only surviving son. Nevertheless, Mary's reputation for unconventional, unwomanly behavior no doubt made it easier for her son to have her declared insane and confined to an asylum. Keeping her there was harder, as Mary vociferously fought the diagnosis of insanity and her forced institutionalization by publicly calling attention to her case.

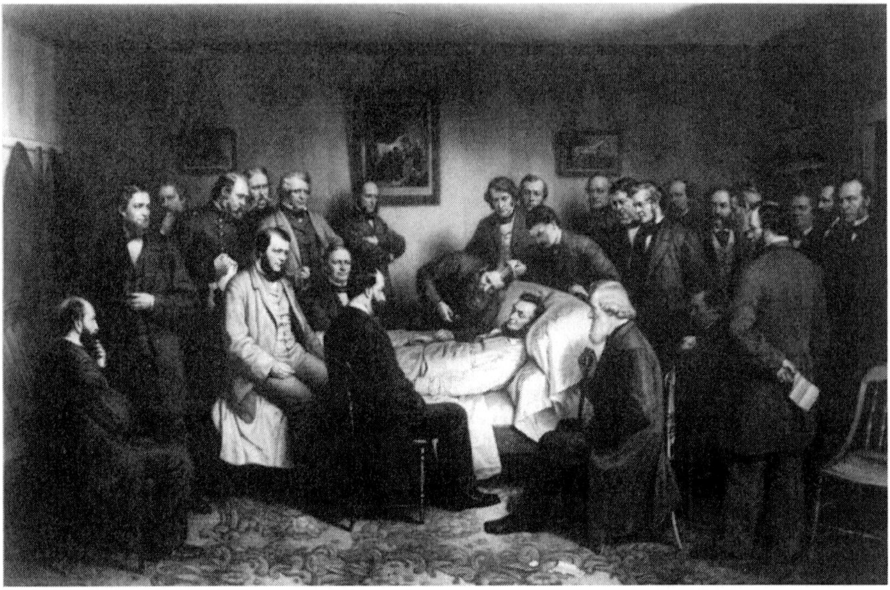

Fig. 4-1. Lithograph by A. H. Ritchie, 1868.

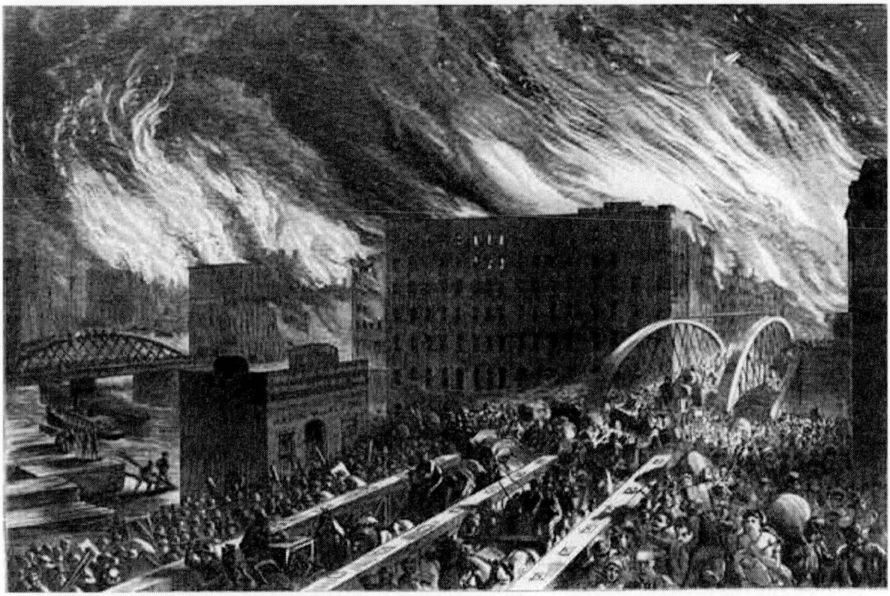

Fig. 4-2. John R. Chapin, *Chicago in Flames—The Rush for Lives Over Randolph Street Bridge*, 1871.

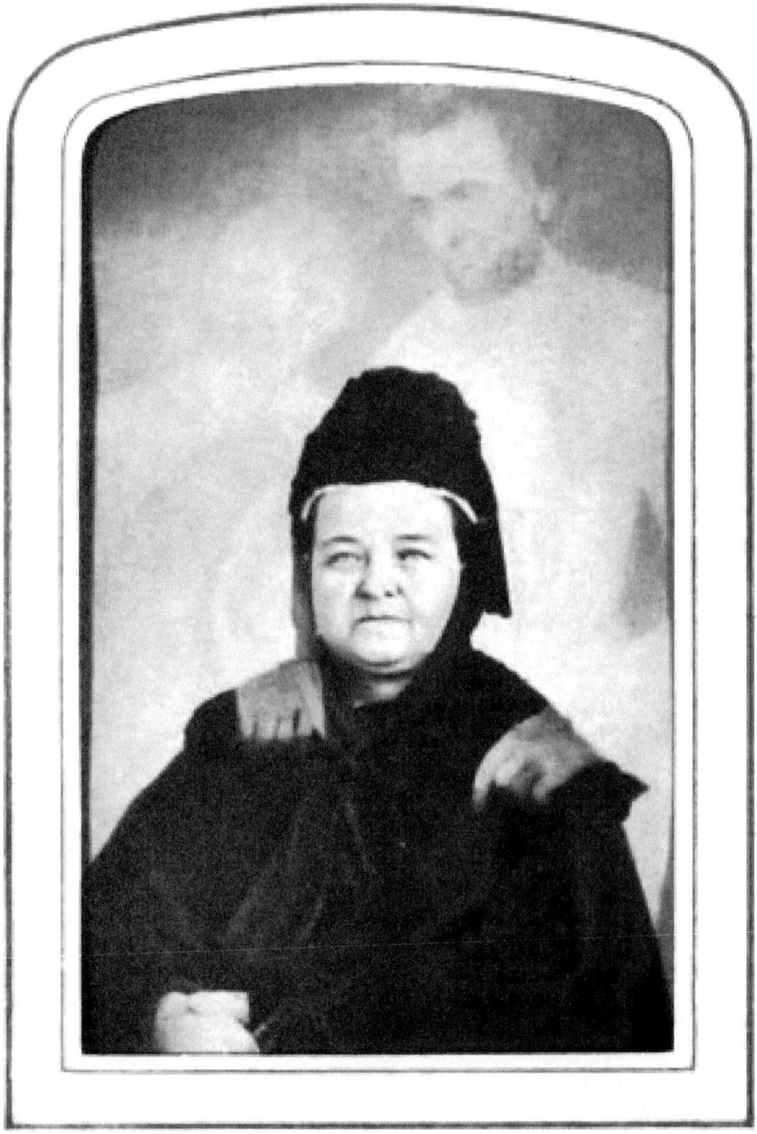

Fig. 4-3. William Mumler's photograph of Mary Lincoln, date unknown.

CHAPTER FIVE

WOMEN IN STRAIGHTJACKETS, MEN IN ARMOR: MALE MANAGEMENT IN *THE WOMAN IN WHITE*

Wilkie Collins's *The Woman in White* is credited with being both the first work of sensational fiction and the most popular. In the preface to the 1860 novel version, Collins acknowledges "the warm welcome my story has met with, in its periodical form, among English and American readers" (644). The warm reception of the work is attributable not only to its ability to elicit thrills in the reader, but to its contemporary subject matter. As Natalie Huffels explains, "While the sensation novel's murderous plots, secret crimes, and alluringly evil villains may still have the power to disturb and fascinate modern readers, Victorian reviewers located the genre's power in its contemporary quality" (42). Collins chose to write his story on a subject that was dominating the headlines during the time of its initial publication: wrongful confinement in insane asylums.

In the nineteenth-century, the English public became obsessed with the threat of wrongful confinement, leading to a series of "lunacy panics." Barbara Leavy explains:

> A year before Collins began writing his novel, public concern about the legal safeguards involving commitment to lunatic asylums had reached a fever pitch. Private pamphlets, the accounts of ex-patients, the sensationalism surrounding some cases that were reported in the newspapers, the continuing agitation from agencies such as the Alleged Lunatics Friends Society—all of these led to the convening of a Parliamentary Select Committee whose hearing ran virtually parallel to the serialization of *The Woman in White*. (105)

The purpose of the committee was to investigate "The Treatment of Lunatics and their Property'" (Sutherland xix). Not only were the results of this investigation published at the same time as the periodical publication of *The Woman in White*, press coverage in general at that time reflected the public's concern over the subject. *Household Words*, the British periodical where *The Woman in White* appeared, featured "frequent accounts of the lunacy reform movement and the development of 'mental science'" (Taylor 53).

Press coverage during the lunacy panics indicates that "[p]ublic anxiety centered on two issues: the technical ease with which a person could be legally incarcerated and kept in a madhouse, and the arbitrary medical basis for diagnosing insanity" (Kurata 43). On August 19, 1858, the *Times* reported: "The fact would appear to be that under existing arrangements any English man or woman may without much difficulty be incarcerated in a Private Lunatic Asylum when not deprived of reason" (qtd. in Leavy 102). While anyone might be wrongly committed, perhaps the person most vulnerable to wrongful confinement in a patriarchal society was a woman who refused to submit to male authority. As Marilyn Kurata explains, "men could deliberately invoke the masculine powers of Victorian medicine and law to disarm, discredit, and confine women who refused to suffer and be still" (43-44).

In *The Woman in White*, Wilkie Collins calls attention to the particular vulnerability of women in a society where wrongful institutionalization was a genuine concern. Inspired by actual cases of rebellious women who were unjustly confined, Collins weaves a tale in which two greedy male villains use the law and medicine as tools to wrongfully imprison women in an insane asylum. While the novel is meant as an exposé on the wrongful institutionalization of women, Collins's message is undermined by the characterization of his female victims as being mentally unstable. Moreover, the story suggests that women are too frail to fight their own battles and are in need of noble knights to shield them from the villains who would confine them. This characterization is not only distorted—since the histories of women wrongfully imprisoned clearly reveal that these women fought their own battles—it reinforces the view that men need to be in control of women, if only for their own protection.

According to John Sutherland, there were three cases of unjust institutionalization that were in the headlines during 1858 (xix). One of these in particular would have been a likely source of inspiration for Collins, as it concerned figures in his own literary circle: Edward and Rosina Bulwer-Lytton. Like the villainous Sir Percival Glyde in *The Woman in White*, Edward Bulwer-Lytton was both a baronet and a "vindictive husband" (Sutherland xx). After he and his wife separated in 1836, Bulwer-Lytton gave his wife only a paltry allowance to live on and denied her access to their children. Indeed, Rosina "was not even allowed to visit her daughter, Emily, on the young girl's deathbed" (Sutherland xx). In retaliation, Rosina tried to shame Bulwer-Lytton by writing novels that satirized him and letters to his London clubs, friends, and the House of Commons (to which he had been elected). Moreover, she also tried to interrupt a performance of a play he had written in which both Charles Dickens and Wilkie Collins were starring (Sutherland xx). The last straw came when Rosina publicly denounced her husband at the nomination meeting for his parliamentary constituency in 1858. This humiliating episode provoked Bulwer-Lytton to find a means of "temporarily gagging and permanently discrediting his worse critic" (Kurata 48).

While only two doctors needed to sign a certificate of insanity, "[a]t least six different physicians provided written opinions that Rosina was insane and should be committed to an asylum, even though none of them had examined her and were basing their diagnosis on a hardly disinterested account of her behavior by a husband who himself had not seen her in two decades" (Kurata 46). Four days after the election, Edward Bulwer-Lytton had two of these doctors call on his wife to issue the certificate of insanity so that she could be committed. However, one of the doctors refused to issue the certificate because he "could not agree upon the alleged unsoundness of her mind" (Kurata 49). Nevertheless, ten days later this same doctor was one of the two medical men who signed the necessary certificate, and Rosina was forcibly taken to an asylum. Marilyn Kurata suggests that the doctors' readiness to commit Rosina was influenced by the fact that her husband was "a rich man, a baronet, a member of Parliament, and a popular novelist" (46), while John Sutherland claims Bulwer-Lytton bribed the doctors to certify his wife (xxi). Regardless, there seems to have been little evidence of insanity or of the premise that Rosina was being institutionalized for her own good. As Kurata explains, "Bulwer-Lytton's conduct throughout this period indicates that his primary concern was neither Rosina's mental condition nor her well-being. The 'evidence' for her insanity was an account of Rosina's consistently hostile behavior since the separation. There was no suggestion that Rosina had suddenly become deranged" (46).

While Bulwer-Lytton was able to persuade six doctors to say that his wife was insane, others were not so easily convinced. Two weeks after Rosina's commitment, the people in the town where she lived called a public meeting to express their outrage at her confinement and demand justice (Kurata 50). The *Somerset County Gazette* reported:

> There is, we say, a firm belief that Lady Lytton is the subject of a horrible and appalling injustice and wrong; that while perfectly sane she has been shut up in a lunatic asylum, merely

> in order that a woman who has, no doubt, been a constant source of annoyance to her husband may be prevented for ever from again giving him similar trouble, or again molesting him in any way. . . . people among whom she has resided during a period of three years—to many of whom she is well and intimately known, and most of whom have had frequent opportunities of seeing her—believe that though sent to an asylum for lunatics, her intellect is perfectly sound. (qtd. in Kurata 51)

The outcry in the local press spread to the London papers, where Bulwer-Lytton and the ministry that had appointed him were severely criticized. Rosina was confined to the asylum for over three weeks while her friends, townspeople, and the press protested her confinement, after which point the Commissioners in Lunacy examined Rosina, pronounced her sane, and released her. According to John Sutherland, "heading the committee was Bryan Waller Procter—the dedicatee of *The Woman in White*" (xxi). Though Rosina Lytton was released, the ease with which she had been committed had disturbing implications. *The Daily Telegraph* reported:

> the lunatic asylums of this country are frequently applied to the same uses as the Bastille, where the Man in the Iron Mask was immured for life because his pretensions were considered dangerous by claimants to estates and title, or perpetrators of unsearched crimes.
>
> But a social question of far more universal importance is connected with the deplorable disclosure in the case of Sir Bulwer Lytton. The baronet's wife may be released from the terrible captivity to which, by the practical confession of her persecutors, she never ought to have been for a moment consigned, and from which we have made no unsuccessful effort to deliver her; but what of humbler persons? What of the domestic victims in whose name no publicity is invoked?" (qtd. in Kurata 52).

These questions struck a nerve in the British public, a nerve that Wilkie Collins decided to exploit by writing a tale of unjust confinement. Upon reading the novel, "Rosina was mightily pleased, and wrote to Collins, congratulating him on his baronet villain. On his part, Bulwer Lytton pronounced *The Woman in White* to be 'vile trash'" (Sutherland xxi).

While the case of Rosina Bulwer-Lytton and the lunacy panic undoubtedly inspired Collins to take up the pen on the subject of wrongful confinement, Lady Lytton's case was too well known and her character too mutinous to provide the proper details for the plot of a popular mystery story. For this, Collins turned to another, more remote case of a woman who had been wrongfully confined. Collins reportedly told a friend that he derived some of his best material, including the plot for *The Woman in White*, from a volume of French crimes that he picked up in a Paris bookstall (Sucksmith 599). According to H. P. Sucksmith, the volume Collins was referring to was Maurice Méjan's *Recueil des Causes Célèbres*, a book he acquired on a trip to Paris with Dickens in 1856 (599). The case that provided Collins with many of the plot details in *The Woman in White* is that of Madame de Douhault, a woman who was institutionalized in France from 1788-1789 (Sucksmith 599).

When Madame de Douhault's father died in 1784, her brother seized the estate, "including some of the inheritance rightfully belonging to his mother and his sister" (Hyder 299). Madame de Douhault set out to recover the rightful property of her mother and herself, and in 1787 she embarked on a trip to Paris for this purpose. En route she stopped at Orleans, where she attempted to stay with a nephew and heir. However, her nephew refused to host Madame de Douhault and instead encouraged her to stay with an acquaintance. The night before her departure for Paris, the wife of this acquaintance offered Madame de Douhault a pinch of snuff, after which she suffered a severe headache and fell asleep. When she awoke several days later, she found herself in the Salpêtrière under a false name. Madame de Douhault had been declared dead, and her estate already liquidated by her brother and heirs. Madame de Douhault's attempts to communicate with the world outside the asylum were thwarted for a time, but she eventually succeeded in smuggling a letter out to a friend, who helped her regain her liberty. (Hyder 299-300) Although she was universally recognized as the supposedly deceased Madame de Douhault, her brother "succeeded in frustrating all her efforts over many years to prove her identity legally and regain her property" (Sucksmith 600). Thus, Collins discovered a true story of a woman whose male heirs had conspired to have her pronounced dead and committed to an asylum so they could inherit her fortune. The case also provided the added benefit of a startling image: when Madame de Douhault was admitted to the asylum she was dressed in white (Sucksmith 600). The idea that a woman could be falsely committed to an asylum by greedy men was exactly the kind of thing the British public was worried about when *The Woman in White* appeared. To make the story more effective, Collins changed the setting to modern England and made the victims of wrongful confinement frail girls rather than a self-sufficient widow.

In *The Woman in White*, Collins clearly feeds the public's fear that the sane are wrongfully confined to insane asylums. He suggests that there are many factors that allow such wrongful confinements to occur: an unjust legal system, self-interested and incompetent doctors, and society's assumption that noblemen are noble. Collins tells the story of two noblemen who imprison two different women in an insane asylum for their own greedy purposes. The asylum not only serves as a way to confine these women, but as a way to discredit them. Once the women have been branded lunatics, anything they say is disbelieved. The experience of being institutionalized actually causes one of the women to lose her mind. The fear that the sane would become insane after being wrongfully confined was another concern that was frequently expressed by the public during the lunacy panics.

Throughout *The Woman in White*, Collins periodically draws attention to the inadequacy of the British legal system in carrying out justice. He begins his tale by proclaiming that "the machinery of the Law" is unfairly affected by "the lubricating influences of oil of gold" (5).[1] According to Collins, the law is not only swayed by wealth, it is actually a servant to the rich: "the Law is still, in certain inevitable cases, the pre-engaged servant of the long purse" (5). Later on, Collins uses the mastermind criminal Count Fosco to expound on the inadequacy of the English legal system: "The machinery [society] has set up for the detection of crime is miserably ineffective—and yet only invent a moral epigram, saying it works well, and you blind everybody to its blunders" (236). He claims, "When the criminal is a resolute, educated, highly-intelligent man, the police, in nine times outs of ten, lose" (236). While Marian and Lady Glyde adamantly oppose Fosco's analysis of the legal system, the ease with which he is able to commit Lady Glyde under another woman's name indicates that he is right. Marian evidently has accepted the problems with the legal system by the time she smuggles her sister out of the asylum illegally, as "any attempt to identify Lady Glyde and to rescue her by legal means, would, even if successful, involve a delay that might be fatal to her sister's intellects, which were shaken already by the horror of the situation to which she had been consigned" (430). Marian's assumption proves correct, for when Walter Hartright presents Lady Glyde's story to a lawyer, he is told "you have not the shadow of a case" (450). Moreover, the lawyer tells Walter that even if he *did* have a case, "the money question always enters into the law question" (454).

The legal system is not the only patriarchal structure that allows women to be wrongfully confined in *The Woman in White*; the medical system is also a culprit. Sir Percival Glyde paid to have Anne Catherick admitted and kept in a private asylum, just as he paid to have two doctors

[1] Whenever page numbers are the only form of citation in the text, I am referring to the primary source.

certify her as insane (132). While this does not necessarily mean that the doctors were in on the conspiracy, it does mean that they were not completely disinterested. Barbara Leavy explains that this was one of the public's major concerns surrounding institutionalization: "so long as asylums were in private hands, then it lay in the interests of proprietors to hold onto their fee-paying patients. Such proprietors, even if they did not actually cooperate with such plots as Sir Percival Glyde's and Count Fosco's, were vulnerable to their machinations" (107). In the book there is no evidence to suggest that the owner of the asylum or the doctors who certified Anne as insane were a part of the conspiracy. Indeed, "Miss Halcombe's own impression was that the owner of the Asylum had not been received into the confidence of Sir Percival and the Count" (427). However, just because these doctors weren't co-conspirators does not mean they were unbiased. Furthermore, Count Fosco himself suggests that the doctors who certified Lady Glyde as insane did so specifically because he wanted them to: "I also procured the services of two gentlemen, who could furnish me with the necessary certificates of lunacy. . . . Both were men whose vigorous minds soared superior to narrow scruples—both were laboring under temporary embarrassments—both believed in ME" (625). These doctors evidently commit Laura because they are more concerned with their own (probably monetary) "embarrassments" than they are with "narrow scruples" of morality. Moreover, their loyalty lies with Fosco, as does the asylum owner's. When Marian speaks to the proprietor of the asylum, "At first, he appeared to be decidedly unwilling to let her communicate with his patient" (427). He only allows Marian to see Laura because she has a letter from Fosco. Upon seeing the letter, "the tone and manner of the owner of the Asylum altered, and he withdrew his objections" (427). These medical men seem to be unquestioning pawns of the noblemen, not disinterested professionals who certify people as insane based on their own expert knowledge of mental illness.

Indeed, Collins does not paint a very favorable portrait of medical doctors even when they are not toadies. The doctor who treats Marian when she becomes ill may be honorable, but he also appears to be incompetent. Although Count Fosco only practices medicine as a hobby, he evidently has knowledge superior to that of the licensed professional. Fosco writes: "All my anxieties were concentrated on Marian's rescue from the hands of the licensed Imbecile who attended her" (618). While the doctor's ignorance prevents him from correctly treating Marian, his pride refuses to allow him to admit any mistakes. Fosco explains: "I had a brief interview with the doctor, at which I protested, in the sacred interests of humanity, against his treatment of Marian's case. He was insolent, as all ignorant people are"

(619). Finally, "the doctor's imbecile treatment of Marian's case had led to the most alarming results. The fever had turned to Typhus" (620). While Marian's illness is physical, we can easily extend the commentary on the incompetence of medical men to include matters of the mind.

While the legal system and medical men are both accomplices in the unfair institutionalization of women in the novel, another unwitting accomplice is society at large. As Fosco explains, "English society . . . is as often the accomplice as it is the enemy of crime" (238). Even the characters who are devoted to the welfare of the victims are in some degree responsible for their institutionalization because they assume that noblemen are, indeed, noble. When Anne Catherick sends a letter to Laura Fairlie warning her against marrying Sir Percival Glyde, Laura's closest friends and advisors accept Glyde's explanation of the letter without question. Mr. Gilmore says that Sir Percival's explanation is "as simple and satisfactory as I had all along anticipated it would be" (131). Gilmore explains that the "high reputation of the gentleman" induced him to believe Glyde (133). Glyde was evidently depending on Gilmore's trust, as he says, "I may fairly expect Mr. Gilmore, as a gentleman, to believe me on my word" (133). However, he invites Marian to ascertain proof of his word by writing to Mrs. Catherick and asking whether she had his approval in institutionalizing her daughter. Marian takes the invitation as an insult, saying: "I hope, Sir Percival, you don't do me the injustice to suppose I distrust you" (133). After receiving Mrs. Catherick's note confirming that she approved her daughter's institutionalization, Marian asks Mr. Gilmore if they have done everything possible to corroborate Glyde's story. Gilmore responds: "'If we are friends of Sir Percival's, who know him and trust him, we have done all, and more than is necessary,' I answered, a little annoyed by this return of her hesitation. 'But if we are enemies who suspect him—'" (139). Again, Marian immediately dismisses the suggestion that she distrusts Glyde as if her suspicion brings dishonor to them both. Later, Mrs. Clements's complete trust of Count Fosco leads her to be the unsuspecting accomplice in Anne's abduction. Anne appears to be the only person in the novel who *does* question the honesty of the nobility. It is only after she ascertains that Walter is "not a man of rank and title" that she exclaims, "Thank God! I may trust *him*" (24).

Of course, Anne is distrustful of noblemen because she has already been wrongfully committed by one. Anne tells Walter little of her situation except: "I have been cruelly used and cruelly wronged" (25). Later on, we discover that Percival Glyde had Anne institutionalized because he believed she knew that he was his father's illegitimate offspring and could, therefore, ruin him by depriving him of his title and property. Though Glyde easily has Anne committed to the asylum, there is no indication that she is actually insane. When Walter first meets her on the road, he observes "There was nothing wild, nothing immoderate in her manner: it was quiet and self-controlled, a little melancholy and a little touched by suspicion" (21). When they meet again and Anne asks Walter if he thinks she should be in an asylum, he tells her: "Certainly not. I am glad you escaped from it; I am glad I helped you" (99). According to Barbara Leavy, "Hartright's feeling that there was no reason for the frightened young woman to be confined would carry much weight at a time when it was also believed that such general impressions were as valid as medical diagnoses" (98). Moreover, Walter is not alone in believing that Anne need not be institutionalized. Anne tells him: "Mrs Clements is like you, she doesn't think I ought to be in the Asylum; and she is glad as you are that I escaped from it" (100).

Just as Percival Glyde has Anne committed to an asylum for selfish reasons, he has his own wife committed out of greed as well. He only marries Laura Fairlie for her fortune. To pay off his debts, Glyde needs a loan from her private fortune that is held in trust for any heirs she might produce. However, when Lady Glyde refuses to sign the papers for the loan, Glyde is more than willing to fake her death and have her committed to an asylum under Anne Catherick's name. Count Fosco is the mastermind behind this plot, as he stands to inherit (via his wife) upon Lady Glyde's death as well. Thus, the story of Laura Glyde's institutionalization is clearly modeled after that of Madame de Douhault. Both women were falsely committed to an asylum by greedy male heirs.

By institutionalizing Anne and Laura, the villains of the story both dispose of and discredit them. After being committed to the asylum, Anne's "hatred and distrust" of the man who placed her there is branded as "insane" and her accusations against him termed evidence of a "marked delusion" (425). Similarly, those in the asylum dismiss Laura's protests about her identity as a "delusion" (425). When committing Laura, Fosco tells the asylum owner that she mistakenly believes she is someone else. Thus, "Fosco nullifies in advance Laura's claims to her true identity, transforming them into proofs of her madness" (Stern 35). When Marian presents Laura to Mr. Fairlie after her escape from the asylum, "the influence of prejudice" prevents him from recognizing her as his niece (438). Being institutionalized casts suspicion over a person which she cannot escape. For this reason, Mrs. Clements admonishes Anne that her confinement "must be kept a secret from everybody" (100). Even after Anne and Laura escape the asylum, to tell their stories is more dangerous to them than it is to the men who had them confined, as they can easily be confined again. Thus, Anne's choice of words is apt when she refers to "[t]he misfortune of my being shut up" (100), as she has been silenced as well as confined.

Being committed to an asylum and branded a lunatic has dire consequences for both women. For Anne, it exacerbates a heart condition that leads to her death. Though Laura does not lose her life, she loses her mind. Afterwards Laura has a "confused and weakened memory" (432). Her experience in the asylum has left her "sorely tried and sadly changed; her beauty faded, her mind clouded" (422). Walter explains: "At the slightest reference to that time, she changed and trembled still; her words became confused; her memory wandered and lost itself as helplessly as ever" (570). As Natalie Huffels notes, the trauma of institutionalizion has left Laura with "severe cognitive impairment" (42). Collins suggests that this horrible outcome is a danger to any sane person who has been wrongfully committed: "she had been under restraint; her identity with Anne Catherick's systematically asserted, and her sanity, from first to last, practically denied. Faculties less delicately balanced, constitutions less tenderly organized, must have suffered under such an ordeal as this. No man could have gone through it, and come out of it unchanged" (436-37). With this suggestion, Collins again draws upon popular fears during the lunacy panic, as both asylum narratives and accounts in the popular press frequently express the concern that wrongful institutionalization can lead to insanity.

While Anne and Laura are both wrongfully confined for financial reasons, they are also both confined directly after they stand up to male authority—specifically Sir Percival. In refusing to obey his commands and behave like obedient women, both are acting contrary to the gender roles society has prescribed for them. They are, of course, punished for their transgressions by being sent to the asylum. Although Marian also defies her proper gender role, she does not openly contradict male authority. She is still punished, though her punishment is physical illness rather than wrongful confinement. Consciously or not, Collins clearly suggests that women who are not passive and submissive will eventually be punished. In contrast with these female rebels stands the Countess, a woman who looks to her husband for guidance in even the smallest matters.

Jenny Taylor suggests that the female in general is an object of "moral management" in the Victorian world: "Moral management becomes the means by which power is exercised and controlled, and repression seems a natural form of domestication. The most extreme form of this is Count Fosco whose control of others is most openly expressed in the moral management of his wife, a formerly wayward woman who is turned into a model asylum patient" (55-56). Marian calls the Count a "magician . . . who has tamed this once wayward Englishwoman" (219). Before her marriage, the Countess used to laugh or scream "as the whims of the moment inclined her" (218). Her husband, however, "transformed her into a civil, silent, unobtrusive woman" (219). The Countess's eyes are "generally turned on her husband, with the look of mute submissive inquiry which we are all familiar with in the eyes of a faithful dog" (219). The Count seems to have tamed his wife just as he has tamed his pets. The Countess had formerly "advocated the Rights of Women—and freedom of female opinion was one of them" (236). Now, however, she does not offer an opinion, but "wait[s] to be instructed" (236). The fact that the Countess follows her husband's instructions in all matters is precisely the reason why he objects to her being a witness when Percival calls upon Lady Glyde to sign the loan paperwork: "we have but one opinion between us, and that is mine" (246). Later on, the Count explains his wife's submissiveness as the duty of an English wife: "I ask, if a woman's marriage obligations, in this country, provide for her opinion of her husband's principles? No! They charge her unreservedly to love, honor, and obey him" (628). As Marilyn Kurata observes, "Fosco's definition of the married Englishwoman's conjugal duties underscores Laura's failure to feel, think, and act as a wife should" (57).

Laura certainly fails to "unreservedly love, honor, and obey" her husband. Thus, she does not conform to the role society has prescribed for her as a woman. When Sir Percival asks Laura to sign the loan paperwork, she refuses, infuriating her husband. He angrily declares that "it is no part of a woman's duty to set her husband at defiance" (250). Though Count Fosco appears to protect Lady Glyde from Sir Percival's wrath, he soon afterwards goes to work concocting the plan that will send this disobedient wife to the asylum. Thus, "The central crisis precipitating Laura's wrongful confinement revolves around her refusal to act like a proper English wife" (Kurata 56). Laura's punishment for refusing to submit to her husband's authority helps to cure her of such rebelliousness. As D. A. Miller observes, "The same internment that renders Laura's body docile, and her mind imbecile, also fits her to incarnate the norm of the submissive Victorian wife" (122).

One need not be a disobedient wife to be wrongfully confined; being a disobedient woman is reason enough. Like Laura, Anne is committed to the asylum shortly after defying Sir Percival's authority. When he commands her to leave the room so he can speak to her mother privately, Anne refuses. In fact, she not only refuses to obey him, she openly threatens him: "Beg my pardon directly . . . or I'll make it the worse for you. I'll let out your Secret. I can ruin you for life, if I choose to open my lips" (549). Of course, Sir Percival will not tolerate being under the thumb of a woman. He immediately persuades Anne's mercenary mother into "shutting her up" by agreeing to confine her to an asylum (550). Thus, "Anne's unwomanly defiance of male authority is punished with incarceration" (Kurata 55).

Although Marian is the most unwomanly female in the novel, her masculine prudence keeps her from openly defying male authority. She knows the consequences would be dire. For this reason, she often suppresses her own natural responses to Sir Percival and Count Fosco and advises her sister Laura to do the same. However, Marian is obviously frustrated with her lack of power as a woman in her society. Eventually, this frustration leads to an attempt to break free of feminine restraints. However, Marian is ultimately punished for overstepping gender boundaries.

Suspecting that Sir Percival and Count Fosco are concocting a diabolical plan against Laura, Marian decides to eavesdrop on their conversation—a most unladylike action. To do so, Marian must shed the feminine clothing that restricts her body just as society restricts her actions: "I took off my silk gown to begin with, because the slightest noise from it . . . might have betrayed me. I next removed the white and cumbersome parts of my underclothing" (326). In discarding her feminine attire, Marian symbolically discards her role as a passive and powerless woman. Her change of clothes allows her to go where women are prohibited: "In my ordinary evening costume, I took up the room of three men at least. In my present dress . . . no man could have passed through the narrowest spaces more easily than I" (326). Because she now has more freedom of movement, Marian is able to eavesdrop on the Count and Percival, an invasion of male space that is most improper for a Victorian lady.

As Marian eavesdrops, she overhears the Count explain to Percival how a man is able to control a woman. A man can either "knock her down" (329), or he can simply refuse to be provoked:

> It holds with animals, it holds with children, and it holds with women, who are nothing but children grown up. Quiet resolution is the one quality the animals, the children, and the women all fail in. If they can once shake this superior quality in their master, they get the better of *him*. If they can never succeed in disturbing it, he gets the better of *them*. (330)

In this speech, the Count makes explicit the connection between animals, children, and women that appears repeatedly throughout the novel. Though he believes that, like animals and children, "all women fail" in resolution, the Count notes that Marian "has the foresight and the resolution of a man" (330). Despite Marian's "manly" resolution, the Count is soon able to manage her. She is manageable not because she has lost her resolution, but because she has been "knock[ed] down" by the forces of nature: she becomes ill after being caught out in the rain while eavesdropping. Marian's loss of control is a direct result of shedding her role as passive woman and invading the privacy of men. Nature itself punishes her. The Count, on the other hand, repeatedly invades Marian's (and Laura's) privacy with impunity by reading letters and diaries and by spying on them. Collins suggests that *women* who overstep their boundaries will inevitably be punished.

Marian's removal to the Elizabethan rooms of the house during her illness suggests a link between her character and that of Queen Elizabeth—a link that Marian would have disdained given her scorn for "that highly overrated woman, Queen Elizabeth" (204). When the housekeeper offers to give Marian a tour of the Elizabethan rooms, Marian declines: "My respect for the integrity of my petticoats and stockings, infinitely exceeds my respect for all the Elizabethan bedrooms in the kingdom" (205). Both her scorn for Queen Elizabeth and her respect for her own feminine attire may indicate that Marian thinks women should remain in the sphere that society has placed them in. It is significant, therefore, that Marian is forced into the Elizabethan rooms after she becomes ill, especially since that illness commences the same night that she sheds her petticoats and stockings and attempts to shed her role of the powerless female.

When Marian oversteps the bounds of womanhood she actually enables Count Fosco and Sir Percival to commit her sister to the asylum. Had she not become ill, they would not have been able to separate the women and exchange Laura's identity for Anne's. Afterwards, Fosco advises Marian with "paternal caution" to submit to her unfortunate circumstances with feminine acquiescence: "Advance no further than you have gone already; . . . threaten nobody" (457). Though Fosco admires Marian's sense and determination, her ostensibly "masculine" attributes pose a threat to the men in the novel. Therefore, Fosco warns her to resign herself to a feminine life of "retirement" and "resignation" in the "modest repose of home" and the "valley of Seclusion" (457). Only such feminine retirement will ensure that she "shall not be molested" (457). Such advice is, by this point, unnecessary. As soon as Walter becomes involved, Marian's role becomes that of assistant rather than leader. Marian is no longer even allowed to speak for herself, as Walter relates her story not in her own words, but in his. Thus, as a result of her own punishment delivered by heaven above, Marian seems to resign herself to the role of the passive female.

Although Marian, Anne, and Laura all defy male authority (whether openly or secretly) and reject the role of passive female at some point in the novel, these acts of defiance are portrayed as unusual rather than typical. In general, women are portrayed as passive, submissive, and content to let men manage their affairs. The first line of the novel tells us, "This is the story of what a Woman's patience can endure, and what a Man's resolution can achieve" (5). Thus, from the beginning we know that the story will demonstrate the passive role of Woman and the aggressive role of Man. The novel portrays women as being too weak to manage their own affairs. Men, then, must manage things for them. Indeed, it is men's duty to control women. While this control takes a malevolent form in the hands of Sir Percival Glyde and Count Fosco, Collins suggests that male management is supposed to have the benevolent purpose of protecting women. The reason Laura is vulnerable to the machinations of Glyde and Fosco in the first place it that her male guardian has failed in his role as manager and protector. After the damsel is delivered to the hands of the villains, she is helpless to defend herself. While Marian attempts to assume the role of protector, as a female she cannot succeed. All seems lost until Walter Hartright—whose heart is in the right place—arrives to defend the damsels in distress, take up the gauntlet against the dastardly villains, and fulfill the quest of establishing Laura's true identity.

Both Anne and Laura are committed to the asylum because they are too weak to defend themselves. Hester Pinhorn says of Anne: "She was but a frail thing to look at, a poor creature! Very little strength, at any time I should say—very little strength" (410). Like Anne, Laura is the stereotypical fragile female. Mrs. Michelson says of her: "She was much too nervous and too delicate in health to bear the anxiety of Miss Halcombe's illness calmly. . . . A more gentle and affectionate lady never lived; but she cried, and she was frightened—two weaknesses which made her entirely unfit to be present in a sick-room" (366). Even in daily life, these women do not seem capable of caring for themselves. Marian plays the role of caretaker for Laura, while Mrs. Clements assumes that role for Anne. When Anne and Laura need protection from men, however, female caretakers are insufficient. Walter Hartright envisions himself as the knight in shining armor to both women. Walter says that he aided Anne when she escaped from the asylum because "[t]he loneliness and helplessness of the woman touched me" (22). He felt compelled by "the natural impulse to assist and spare" the "forlorn woman" he met on the road to London in the middle of the night (22-23). Just as he assists Anne in eluding her captors, Walter assists Laura in regaining her identity. Actually, he regains Laura's identity for her, as "she is utterly incapable of assisting the assertion of her own case" (574). Walter presumes Laura is too feeble to even be made aware of the battle that he is fighting on her behalf: "the wrong that had been inflicted on her, if mortal means could grapple it, must be redressed without her knowledge and without her help" (444).

Although Walter plays the role of benevolent knight in his management of Laura's affairs, the control he assumes is just one form of the control all men seem to think it is their prerogative to assert over women in the novel. Walter alludes to the potentially menacing nature this control can assume when he describes Anne as being "utterly and helplessly at my mercy" (23), and Anne is certainly aware of it herself when she pleads with Walter "not to interfere with me" (22). While Walter complies with this request, he later regrets his "ill-considered promise to leave her free to act as she pleased" (28), suggesting that he had the right to control her actions. Walter worries that he has "cast loose on the whole wide world of London an unfortunate creature, whose actions it was my duty, and every man's duty, mercifully to control" (29). He asks himself if "she was still capable of controlling her own actions" (29), but one must wonder if Victorian men ever considered women to be capable of controlling their own actions.

Walter is unsure as to whether he has exerted the right type of control over Anne by rescuing her from her captors rather than capturing her himself. After all, "[t]hanks to his help, Anne eludes a manifold of male guardians: the turnpike man at the entry gate of the city; the two men from the Asylum including its director; the policeman who, significantly, is assumed to be at their disposal; and even Walter himself, who puts her into a cab, destination unknown" (Miller 111). Either Walter has performed his duty by helping a woman escape wrongful confinement or he has neglected his duty by allowing an insane woman to escape male control. Whether the control exerted is malevolent or benevolent depends on the sanity of the woman. Sir Percival pretends to be motivated by benevolence by proclaiming Anne to be insane and declaring, "It is a duty we all owe to the poor creature to trace her" (134). Percival not only acts as if he has "done his duty to the unhappy young woman, by instructing his solicitor to spare no expense in tracing her, and in restoring her once more to medical care," he also claims "he was only anxious to do his duty towards Miss Fairlie and towards her family, in the same plain, straightforward way" (132). Indeed, by shrouding his actions under the guise of "duty," Sir Percival is able to exert a malevolent form of control over both women by confining them to the asylum.

While Sir Percival disguises his malevolent management of women under the cloak of "duty," Mr. Fairlie utterly neglects his duty to protect his niece and manage her affairs—a duty that he should be honor-bound to fulfill not just as the male head of the family, but as her legal guardian. Mr. Fairlie is responsible for arranging Laura's marriage to Sir

Percival Glyde, but he never seems to take this responsibility seriously, despite the fact that he is placing his niece's life in another man's hands. As a guardian and as a man, he fails in the role of female-protector because he is far more concerned with himself than he is with his niece. When the family lawyer goes to see Mr. Fairlie regarding concerns he has about the marriage contract,

> His talk was to the same purpose as usual—all about himself and his ailments. . . . The moment I tried to speak of the business that had brought me to the house, he shut his eyes and said that I 'upset' him. I persisted in upsetting him by returning again and again to the subject. All I could ascertain was that he looked on his niece's marriage as a settled thing . . . and that he should be personally rejoiced when the worry of it was over. (129-30).

Mr. Fairlie wanted to "limit his share in the business, as guardian, to saying, Yes, at the right moment" (130). For this reason, he lets Glyde determine the terms of the marriage. The lawyer repeatedly urges Mr. Fairlie to refuse to give up Laura's right to dispose of her own money in the marriage contract, but Mr. Fairlie answers "in the interests of peace and quietness, positively No!" (162). He lets Glyde choose the marriage day, despite Marian's protests, allowing Glyde to fix on a date before Laura comes of age so that she has no say in the terms of the marriage contract herself. Mr. Fairlie cannot even bother to tell Laura about the arrangements he agrees to; instead, he has Marian deliver the news. Marian bitterly notes Mr. Fairlie's neglect of his duty, saying: "he seemed perfectly satisfied, so far, with having simply shifted one more family responsibility from his own shoulders to mine" (182). Indeed, if he had been a proper male guardian Marian likely would not have felt the need to step outside her female role.

After the marriage takes place and Laura is in need of male protection from her husband, it is Mr. Fairlie's responsibility to provide that protection. Marian tells Laura: "Your uncle is your nearest male relative, and the head of the family. He must and shall interfere" (307). When Laura expresses her disbelief that he will take the trouble, Marian responds: "your uncle is a weak, selfish, worldly man, I know. . . . But he will do anything to pamper his own indolence and secure his own quiet. Let me only persuade him that his interference, at this moment, will save him inevitable trouble and wretchedness and responsibility hereafter, and he will bestir himself for his own sake" (307). When Mr. Fairlie gets a letter from Marian explaining the conjugal troubles of his niece, he is predictably only worried about himself: "If I opened Limmeridge House as an asylum to Lady Glyde, what security had I against Sir Percival Glyde's following her here, in a state of violent resentment against *me* for harbouring his wife?" (353). As a result of his selfishness, Mr. Fairlie invites Marian to come without Laura. His invitation receives no response, but instead of fearing the meaning of the silence he relishes it: "Her unexpected absence did me amazing good" (354). After Mr. Fairlie learns that Marian's lack of response is due to serious illness, he is worried about himself rather than her, fearing that the messenger may have brought an infectious disease with him (358). Although Laura's maid told Mr. Fairlie of how Marian had charged her with delivering letters to both Mr. Fairlie and the lawyer, and how she seems to have been drugged by Madame Fosco while in possession of those letters, Mr. Fairlie blinds himself to the implications when the lawyer writes and asks if he knows why Marian would have sent him a blank sheet of paper: "What the deuce should I know about it? Why alarm *me* as well as himself? I wrote back to that effect" (354). It is Mr. Fairlie's repeated, selfish neglect of his duty to protect his niece that allows Sir Percival Glyde and Count Fosco to succeed in the plot to wrongfully confine her.

Collins condemns Mr. Fairlie's neglect of "duty" just as he condemns Percival's abuse of the term. Meanwhile, Walter is utterly confused as to what his duty is. The real trouble—which Collins seems to ignore—is the fact that men in the novel see it as their duty to manage women. Even Walter's benevolent management of Laura is just another form of the same control that Percival and Fosco use to incarcerate her.

In addition to reinforcing the Victorian view that it is men's responsibility to manage women (if only for benevolent purposes), Collins also undermines his intended message about the wrongful confinement of women by associating mental and nervous illnesses with femininity. While neither Anne nor Laura seems to belong in an insane asylum, both are portrayed as mentally unstable even before their confinements. And although there is a male character in the novel who suffers from a nervous illness, he is mockingly portrayed as effeminate. By reinforcing the stereotypical cultural associations between mental illness and femininity, Collins unconsciously strengthens the justification for female institutionalization that his novel intends to question.

Although Percival Glyde had Anne confined to a madhouse for self-interested reasons, she does not seem entirely stable. Walter Hartright tells us that until he found out Anne had escaped from an asylum, "the idea of absolute insanity which we all associate with the very name of an Asylum, had, I can honestly declare, never occurred to me, in connexion with her" (28). However, Anne's manner does suggest "either that she was naturally flighty and unsettled, or that some recent shock of terror had disturbed the balance of her faculties" (28). Furthermore, upon reading

Anne's letter to Laura, Walter and Marian agree that it seems as if it were written by "'a woman whose mind must be—' 'Deranged'" (80). Of course, Anne's derangement can in some degree be attributed to the trauma of institutionalization. When Walter refers to her time in the asylum, Anne's face "became suddenly darkened by an expression of maniacally intense hatred and fear, which communicated a wild, unnatural force to every feature. Her eyes dilated in the dim evening light, like the eyes of a wild animal" (104). She tells Walter: "I shall lose myself if you talk of that" (104). When Walter mentions the name of Sir Percival Glyde, "a scream burst from her that rang through the churchyard and made my heart leap in me with the terror of it. The dark deformity of the expression which had just left her face, lowered on it once more, with doubled and trebled intensity" (105).

While Anne's startling moments of temporary derangement are triggered when Walter mentions the asylum or the man who placed her there, she was evidently mentally unstable long before her institutionalization. Percival tells Fosco: "Fancy my wife, after a bad illness, with a touch of something wrong in her head—and there is Anne Catherick for you" (339). He calls Anne "just mad enough to be shut up, and just sane enough to ruin me when she's at large" (337). Anne's mother confirms the view that her daughter was mentally unsound, saying "Anne had been more than usually crazy and queer" the year she was locked up (549). Even Mrs. Clements, Anne's caretaker, says that Anne was "always queer, with her whims and her ways, ever since I can remember her. Harmless, though—as harmless, poor soul, as a child" (94).

At times Anne is described as "crazy," but at other times she is described as being mentally disabled. Mrs. Catherick says that her daughter was "always weak in the head" (547). Mrs. Fairlie wrote about Anne as a child: "the poor little thing's intellect is not developed as it ought to be at her age. . . . her unusual slowness in acquiring ideas implies an unusual tenacity in keeping them, when they are once received into her mind" (58-59). Similarly, Mrs. Catherick says of Anne: "When she *had* got a notion once fixed in her mind she was, like other half-witted people, as obstinate as a mule in keeping it" (548). The problem began when Percival Glyde told Mrs. Catherick to "[t]urn the idiot out" so they could speak privately (549). Mrs. Catherick explains: "that word, 'idiot,' upset her in a moment" (549). Anne pretends to know Glyde's secret "out of crazy spite against him" (550). Mrs. Catherick tries to explain to Glyde that her daughter doesn't really know anything: "I referred him to other queer ways of hers, and to his own experience of the vagaries of half-witted people" (550). However, Glyde insists on shutting Anne up in the asylum. According to Mrs.

Catherick, "The only drawback of putting her under restraint was a very slight one. We merely turned her empty boast about knowing the Secret, into a fixed delusion" (551).

The line between mental illness and mental handicap is blurred in the book, reflecting a general confusion in society about how to categorize "idiots." John Conolly,

> the man whom *Household Words* had called 'the highest living authority' on insanity was quite explicit in his belief that among those patients improperly put in asylums, not necessarily because of malice but because of ignorance on the part of his own profession, were what his age called 'idiots'—people not so much insane but mentally retarded or in other ways deficient. (Leavy 111)

Anne is evidently what would have been described as an "idiot," and as such she does not belong in an asylum. However, at various points in the novel her behavior is described as being "deranged" or "crazy." The mental instability that such terms suggest undermines the idea that she has been sent to the asylum unjustly.

Unlike Anne, Laura is never described as "crazy" or "deranged," and her institutionalization seems even more obviously wrongful given that she was sent to the asylum under a false name. However, Laura is not the picture of mental health either. When Walter first meets Marian, she tells him: "My sister is in her own room, nursing that essentially feminine malady, a slight headache" (33). While her headache may be dismissed as a temporary physical malady, there is the suggestion throughout the novel that she suffers from something more. When Walter meets Laura, he notes that despite the charm of her face there appears to be "something wanting. . . . Something wanting, something wanting—and where it was, and what it was, I could not say" (50-51). Mr. Gilmore describes Laura as looking "pale and sad" (142), and notes that "her fingers had a restless habit, which I remembered in her as a child, of always playing with the first thing that came to hand" (143). Furthermore, "Her eyes moved uneasily from object to object in the room" (143). Taken together, these are symptoms of a nervous illness. Indeed, she is repeatedly described as suffering from nerves. Fosco and Percival are able to separate Laura and Marian because "Lady Glyde was confined to her room by nervous illness" (621). Like Walter, Marian thinks it necessary to shield Laura from potentially disturbing news because it may be too much for her nerves, but Marian thinks such precautions are necessary even before Laura's confinement and when the news seemingly has nothing to do with her. When Walter tells

Marian of meeting the woman in white on the road, Marian responds: "You had better not speak of it yet to Mr Fairlie, or to my sister. . . . They are both of them . . . in widely different ways, rather nervous and sensitive; and you would only fidget one and alarm the other to no purpose" (36).

As D.A. Miller notes, "Of the novel's three characters who seem 'born' nervous, two are women (Anne and Laura) and the third, Mr. Fairlie, an effeminate" (110). Indeed, Mr. Fairlie's nervous illness and his effeminacy are inextricably linked:

> His beardless face was thin, worn, and transparently pale. . . . His feet were effeminately small, and were clad in buff-coloured silk stockings, and little womanish bronze-leather slippers. Two rings adorned his white delicate hands. . . . Upon the whole, he had a frail, languidly-fretful, over-refined look—something singularly and unpleasantly delicate in its association with a man. (40)

Mr. Fairlie says of himself, "I am nothing but a bundle of nerves dressed up to look like a man" (356), though the disguise is not very convincing. He describes himself as being in a "state of nervous wretchedness" and says that he is "shattered by my miserable health" (345). Fosco agrees that "this gentleman was equally feeble in mind and body" (620). Though Mr. Fairlie is an invalid, the nature of his malady is never fully understood. Marian tells Walter, "I don't know what is the matter with him, and the doctors don't know what is the matter with him, and he doesn't know himself what is the matter with him. We all say it's on the nerves, and we none of us know what we mean when we say it" (34).

While nervousness in Anne and Laura seems both natural and pitiable, Collins portrays this same trait as both unnatural and repulsive in a man. Walter tells us, "my sympathies shut themselves up resolutely at the first sight of Mr Fairlie" (40), and it is obvious that the reader is supposed to despise Mr. Fairlie as well. His first and last concern is always himself, and he is constantly making ludicrous excuses and demands in the name of his illness: "In the wretched state of my nerves, movement of any kind is exquisitely painful to me" (40); "In the wretched state of my nerves, loud sound of any kind is indescribable torture to me" (40); "In the wretched state of my nerves, exertion of any kind is unspeakably disagreeable to me" (41); "You have no idea of the tortures I should suffer, Mr Hartright, if Louis dropped that portfolio" (42); "Do you mind my closing my eyes while you speak? Even this light is too much for them" (43); "Gently with the curtains please—the slightest noise from them goes through me like a knife" (44).

Mr. Fairlie is universally the subject of scorn, and the text suggests that his illness is imaginary rather than real.

The negative connotation surrounding Mr. Fairlie's nervous illness stands in marked contrast to the treatment of Anne and Laura's because he is male instead of female. Mr. Fairlie's symptoms are consistent with a diagnosis of hypochondriasis, a mental illness that was associated with men rather than women. This nineteenth-century category of male illness is the root of our modern conception of the hypochondriac. In the Victorian world, mental and nervous illnesses were typically associated with femininity.[2] Thus, it was considered natural that Anne and Laura suffer from such female maladies, whereas a man suffering from a similar disorder is portrayed as a freak of nature. For this reason, Mr. Fairlie is derided for his effeminacy and nearly disqualified from being a man. Indeed, if he were a proper man he would have performed his role of manager and protector of women more suitably. While Mr. Fairlie may be scorned by everyone he meets—characters and readers alike—because he is a man suffering from a female malady, his sex gives him an advantage over the more sympathetically portrayed female sufferers: he is never confined to an insane asylum.

The Woman in White both fed off and fueled the lunacy panic gripping England at the time of its original publication. The British public was suspicious of the medical basis for diagnosing insanity and concerned that the legal system allowed people to be wrongfully institutionalized. This was a topic that Collins would return to again and again. According to Richard Currie, Collins published a total of five novels that "critically explore how Victorian psychiatry determined insanity, made diagnoses and classified varieties of mental illness" (18). When Collins took up the subject of wrongful confinement in *The Woman in White*, he focused on the vulnerability of women in a patriarchal society.[3] Inspired by true stories in which women were wrongfully confined, *The Woman in White* tells the tale of two women who are unjustly institutionalized as punishment for defying male authority.

Although the novel is clearly an exposé on wrongful confinement—specifically the wrongful confinement of women—the power of Collins's message is undercut by his portrayal of the female victims as being mentally

[2] While nervous illnesses were generally associated with femininity, "[n]o doctor implied that signs of nervous disorder were apparent only in women in nineteenth-century America, and the historian should not overlook this evidence. The fact remains, nonetheless, that to some extent the diagnosis, and to a greater extent the treatment by doctors of these symptoms in women, was different from their interpretation of the same signs in men" (Wood 28).

[3] Collins had a reputation as a radical thinker and social critic.

unstable. Of course, confinement in an asylum is not warranted in all cases of mental illness. However, the fact that the female characters who are unjustly confined suffer from some degree of mental illness only strengthens the cultural association between women and madness that made women particularly vulnerable to unjust incarceration in the first place. Furthermore, Collins reinforces the Victorian view that it is men's responsibility to manage women. Both female victims in the novel are too weak to take care of themselves, and both need a knight in shining armor to rescue them from the machinations of the evil villains. However, this knight's chivalrous management of female affairs is only another form of the same control that the villains use to incarcerate them.

CHAPTER SIX

THE VICTORIAN SECRET: DISPOSING OF DEVIANTS LIKE LADY AUDLEY

Many critics have claimed that *Lady Audley's Secret* is a subversive text. While some critics focus on how the text exposes the artificiality of Victorian social norms, others focus on the punishment that attends deviating from them. In "Strong Women and Feeble Men: Upsetting Gender Stereotypes in Mary Elizabeth Braddon's *Lady Audley's Secret*," Herbert Klein argues that the novel is a critique of Victorian gender stereotypes. Both Klein and Pamela Gilbert suggest that women who actively transgress their gender role in Victorian society are punished. In "Madness and Civilization: Generic Opposition in Mary Elizabeth Braddon's *Lady Audley's Secret*," Gilbert focuses on how society silences the voices of those who deviate from the dominant masculine narrative. Like Gilbert, Jill Matus focuses on how the Other is silenced in Victorian society. In "Disclosure as 'Cover-up': The Discourse of Madness in *Lady Audley's Secret*," Matus explains how madness is used to label deviant behavior. These critics laud the subversive nature of the novel, and they interpret Lady Audley's institutionalization as a metaphor for the oppression of the disempowered Other who deviates from societal norms. However, by identifying Lady Audley's incarceration as a metaphor and generalizing about the patriarchal suppression of deviant women, these critics neglect the specific historical circumstances that prompted the story: stories of sane people incarcerated in asylums.

Since the early eighteenth century, the English public was concerned that sane people were being confined in insane asylums. The Madhouse Act of 1774 tried to put an end to this concern by requiring a medical certification of insanity for each admitted patient. Despite this and subsequent reforms, wrongful incarcerations continued into the Victorian era, and public anxiety erupted in a series of lunacy panics. Several works of non-fiction were released by former inmates testifying to wrongful incarceration, and newspapers frequently "printed articles demanding inquiries and suggesting reforms" (McCandless 342). These tales inspired several sensational novels—Henry Cockton's *Valentine Vox* (1840), Wilkie Collins's *The Woman in White* (1860), and Charles Reade's *Hard Cash* (1863). Although *Lady Audley's Secret* (1862) was also published shortly after an incarceration scare, critics have not traditionally examined the novel in this historical context. While critics have understood Lady Audley's incarceration as punishment for her deviant behavior, they have generally ignored the fact that she was incarcerated in an insane asylum rather than a prison. And although Jill Matus has linked deviancy to madness in *Lady Audley's Secret*, she stubbornly refuses to acknowledge the lunacy panic as an inspiration for the novel. However, examining Braddon's book in relation to the lunacy panic drastically changes the way we understand the text. Such an examination reveals that Braddon does not actually condemn the doctors who label deviant people insane. Instead, she sympathizes with their intentions to keep society safe from such deviants.

Although Lady Audley claims that madness is responsible for her deviance, there is little justification for such a diagnosis. While some Victorian doctors equated madness with deviance in a condition called moral insanity, the doctor who examines Lady Audley makes no allusion to it. On the contrary, Dr. Mosgrave tells Robert: "I do not believe that she is mad" (248). He explains that "there is no evidence of madness in anything she has done" (248). Dr. Mosgrave determines that Lady Audley is sane largely because there are logical reasons for her actions: "She ran away from her home, because it was not a pleasant one and she left in the hope of finding a better. There is no madness in that. She committed the crime of bigamy, because by that crime she obtained fortune and position. There is no madness there" (248). While Lady Audley might have behaved immorally in abandoning her child and committing bigamy, she had clear motives. As Roger Smith explains, motives are evidence of sanity (122). Lady Audley's sanity is also indicated by her rational powers of calculation: "When she found herself in a desperate position, she did not grow desperate. She employed intelligent means, and she carried out a conspiracy which required coolness and deliberation in its execution. There is no madness in that" (248). Lady Audley's ability to reason under pressure is particularly indicative of a strong mind, not a weak one. Dr. Mosgrave concludes: "I do not think there is any proof of insanity in the story you have told me. I do not think any jury in England would accept the plea of insanity in such a case as this" (248). Dr. Mosgrave's verdict is clear: though she is a deviant, Lady Audley is also sane.

In order to persuade Dr. Mosgrave to certify Lady Audley as insane, Robert repeatedly draws upon Dr. Mosgrave's sense of duty to society. When Robert appeals to Dr. Mosgrave to reconsider his diagnosis of Lady Audley, Robert assures him: "I do not ask you to do any wrong to society; but I ask you to save our stainless name from degradation and shame" (249). Robert then explains that he suspects Lady Audley of killing her first husband and "conclude[s] with an earnest appeal to the physician's best feelings" (249). Dr. Mosgrave agrees to a brief interview with Lady Audley, after which he declares: "The lady is not mad; but she has the hereditary taint in her blood. She has the cunning of madness, with the prudence of intelligence. I will tell you what she is, Mr. Audley. She is dangerous!" (249). Although Dr. Mosgrave still insists that "The Lady is not mad," he finally agrees to certify that she is mad because "She is dangerous!" However, Dr. Mosgrave does not falsify Lady Audley's commitment papers out of any dishonorable motives. He does so because he considers her a threat to the society. Moreover, the decision is evidently one that he wrestles with. He paces the room as he explains his reasoning: "This Mr. George Talboys has disappeared, but you have no evidence of his death. If you could produce evidence of his death, you could produce no evidence against this lady, beyond the one fact that she had a powerful motive for getting rid of him. No jury in the United Kingdom would condemn her upon such evidence as that" (250). Because Lady Audley cannot be imprisoned via a court of law, she must be imprisoned by other means. Dr. Mosgrave tells Robert: "you cannot expect me to condone one of the worst offenses against society. If I saw adequate reason for believing that a murder had been committed by this woman, I should refuse to assist you in smuggling her away out of reach of justice, although the honor of a hundred noble families might be saved by my doing so. But I do not see adequate reason for your suspicions; and I will do my best to help you" (250). Although Robert's primary objective is preserving the family honor, Dr. Mosgrave repeatedly insists that he does not share that concern. Could Lady Audley be convicted in court, Dr. Mosgrave would not declare her insane. However, he is willing to certify her because he believes she would not be convicted in a court of law and is a danger to society if left free.

Dr. Mosgrave's decision to certify Lady Audley despite her sanity is indicative of the power that doctors could wield for good or evil in nineteenth-century England. While it is possible to read Dr. Mosgrave as a negative portrayal of how mind-doctors assumed a role of moral authority, falsely imprisoned sane people, and reinforced the patriarchy, it is easier to read him as a positive defense of mind-doctors and a justification for how and why the institutionalization of sane people might occur. Braddon vividly portrays Dr. Mosgrave as a man struggling with a serious ethical dilemma that many doctors must have faced when diagnosing someone in nineteenth-century England: "If they declared him insane and confined him, and a jury later disagreed with a diagnosis, people would accuse them of nefarious behavior; if they pronounced him sane and left him at large, and he later committed an outrage, the public would condemn them as incompetent" (McCandless 348). Dr. Mosgrave ultimately decides that committing a sane woman to an asylum is the lesser evil in Lady Audley's case: "Whatever crimes she may have committed she will be able to commit no more. . . . But as a physiologist and as an honest man, I believe you could do no better service than by doing this: for physiology is a lie if the woman I saw ten minutes ago is a woman to be trusted at large," he tells Robert (250-51). Robert appears to adopt Dr. Mosgrave's attitude, as his motives shift from preserving family honor to preserving the safety of society. Before he leaves her at the asylum, Robert tells Lady Audley that he would be "a traitor to society had I suffered you to remain at liberty" (256), and he "impressed upon Monsieur Val, that under no circumstances was she to be permitted to leave the house and grounds" (255). Although the decision to imprison Lady Audley at a *maison de santé* in Belgium is certainly a violation of her rights, it also eliminates a threat to society at large.

The decision to send Lady Audley to a Belgian *maison de santé* is an important one, especially since the lunacy panic revolved around wrongful imprisonment within England. By exporting Lady Audley to a foreign country for her institutionalization, Braddon drew attention to the fact that the lunacy laws in England were stricter than they were in Belgium. After the Madhouse Act of 1828, two medical doctors were required to sign a certificate of commitment in England. The laws in Belgium and France only required the certification of one doctor, so long as that doctor was unconnected to the asylum. Thus, Lady Audley is committed to the asylum in Villebrumeuse upon the word of Dr. Mosgrave alone. In England, Robert would have needed another doctor willing to sign Lady Audley's commitment papers in addition to Dr. Mosgrave. In contrast, the superintendent at Villebrumeuse doesn't even examine Lady Audley when she is admitted. He sycophantically tells Robert that there was "nothing under heaven which he would not strive to accomplish for him, as the friend of his acquaintance, so very much distinguished, the English doctor. Dr. Mosgrave's letter had given him a brief synopsis of the case . . . and he was quite prepared to undertake the care of the charming and very interesting Madam" (254). Apart from the "brief synopsis" Dr. Mosgrave provides, the superintendent knows nothing about Lady Audley at all. Robert provides no specifics about her, and their conversation only "occupied about a quarter of an hour" (255). Although Robert "had to see all manner or important personages; and to take numerous oaths; and to exhibit the English physician's letter; and to go through much ceremony of signing and countersigning" before taking Lady

Audley to the asylum (252), her institutionalization would have been impossible in England with only the certificate of one doctor and the say-so of a nephew. Perhaps Lady Audley is shrewdly referring to the ease with which a person can be committed in a foreign asylum when she tells Robert that "they manage these things better in France" (254).

In addition to an examination of Lady Audley's commitment, an examination of the characters' economic motives also reveals that the novel is a reaction against the recent lunacy panic. As Peter McCandless explains, "In the minds of many Victorians money was at the root of the problem of wrongful confinement" (343). In many of the cases in the press, sane people were confined so that relatives could control their money or property. As a result, the British public was largely under the impression that sane people were placed in insane asylums as a result of greedy malevolence. Therefore, if Braddon were suggesting that sane people were incarcerated unjustly, she would probably have made the motivation for Lady Audley's confinement a monetary one, as did the authors of the other three Victorian novels about the institutionalization of sane people. However, money is most decidedly *not* the motive for institutionalizing Lady Audley. As I have already shown, both Robert Audley and Dr. Mosgrave decide to commit Lady Audley to an insane ayslum because they consider her to be a threat to society. Thus, *Lady Audley's Secret* provides a fairly positive assessment of the lunacy laws in England, as Braddon wrote a story in which "the men who certified and confined lunatics did so because they believed that it was in the best interests of society and the individuals concerned" (McCandless 357). Even when Dr. Mosgrave and Robert decide to bend the rules to commit a sane criminal, they have to do so in another country because the laws of England are stricter. The fact that Dr. Mosgrave and Robert Audley are motivated by the desire to protect society rather than their pocketbooks is an indication that Braddon's book is not intended as an exposé about unjust confinement, but a reaction against such stories.

Although those who incarcerate Lady Audley are not motivated by money, Lady Audley is. When Sir Michael proposes to Lady Audley and tells her that she should not accept him for monetary reasons, Lucy replies: "I *cannot* be disinterested; I cannot be blind to the advantages to such an alliance. I cannot, I cannot!" (8). While her honesty here is admirable and her concern for money understandable, Lady Audley's preoccupation with money is an indication that her motives are not pure. Even as a child, she schemes about how to catch a "rich suitor" and become "more successful in the world's great lottery than my companions" (231). She only loves her first husband "as long his money lasted" (232), and after his money runs out she "upbraided George Talboys for his cruelty and in having allied a helpless girl to poverty and misery" (232). She gladly escapes that marriage for another with a richer man and is willing to commit murder rather than surrender her riches. While we can sympathize with Lady Audley's fear of poverty, her willingness to kill others in order to maintain her elevated position emphasizes her immorality. Additionally, her plot to have Robert Audley wrongly institutionalized to protect her own wealth makes her more akin to the villain of an incarceration scheme than the victim.

Because *Lady Audley's Secret* was written in the immediate aftermath of widespread panic over the incarceration of sane people in insane asylums, Lady Audley's fate needs to be considered with this historical context in mind. By her own admission, Braddon's book was a response to Wilkie Collins's *The Woman in White* (N. Donaldson vii), the sensational novel most commonly linked to the incarceration scare. While Collins's heroine is a frail, innocent woman in need of a savior, Braddon's is a dangerous woman who needs to be institutionalized for the safety of society. Both the depiction of Lady Audley's commitment and the motives of the characters in the novel indicate that Braddon's story is a reaction against the lunacy panic rather than another story fueling that panic. *Lady Audley's Secret* is not an exposé deploring the wrongful incarceration of social deviants. Braddon rather sympathizes with the doctors who try to protect society from such deviants. Braddon's response to the lunacy panic is likely influenced by the experiences of those close to her, specifically John Maxwell and Edward Bulwer-Lytton. Braddon lived with Maxwell for fourteen years and had five children with him before they could be married, as he already had a wife living in a mental institution. Due to her own situation, Braddon may have been sensitive about accusations regarding the wrongful institutionalization of family members. In addition, the novel was dedicated to her mentor and friend, Edward Bulwer-Lytton, a man who had his own wife incarcerated just a few years before the novel's publication.

Rosina and Edward Bulwer-Lytton separated in 1836. However, Rosina claimed that Edward did not provide her with enough money to survive, so she decided to publicly expose him at the Hertford election, where he was running for parliament, in 1858. He responded by having her committed to a private madhouse. After three weeks of public outrage, Rosina was released. While public sympathy was generally in favor of Lady Lytton's release, Braddon's relationship to Bulwer-Lytton may have skewed her opinion of the fiasco. Although the circumstances surrounding the incarceration of Lady Lytton and Lady Audley are wildly different, there are similarities worth noting. Money was, ultimately, what fueled both Lady Lytton and Lady Audley. Lady Lytton ended up in the asylum because she was trying to extort money from her husband. Lady Audley married for money and ended up in the asylum because she would do anything to keep it. By altering the circumstances of the incarceration, Braddon flips the typical view that those enforcing institutionalization were the greedy ones. This role reversal is also hinted at in the final chapter of the book, where Clara Talboys refers to her brother—not Lady Audley—as having a "blighted life" because of his wife (282). *A Blighted Life* is the title of Rosina Bulwer Lytton's incarceration tale. Although Rosina Bulwer Lytton's memoir was not published until 1880, the manuscript had been lying around for years before its publication, and it would not be surprising if Braddon was aware of its title. Furthermore, both Lady Lytton and Lady Audley were confined in rather lush quarters, though they were nonetheless "buried alive" due to their lack of liberty.

Unlike other critics, Jill Matus acknowledges similarities between *Lady Audley's Secret* and the story of Rosina Bulwer Lytton. While Matus points out that Edward Bulwer-Lytton had his wife confined to a madhouse just a few years prior to the novel's publication, she does not believe that Lytton's story inspired Braddon's. If Braddon had intended to expose the wrongful institutionalization of women, Matus suggests, she would have chosen a protagonist who was "clearly sane" and innocent (349). Instead, Matus argues that Braddon's story is a "metaphorical" portrayal of the hegemony's suppression of the Other rather than an explicit exposé of the incarceration of sane women in insane asylums (352). There are a couple of problems with Matus's argument. Firstly, if Braddon intended to depict how non-conformists were punished in society—regardless of whether institutionalization is taken to be a metaphorical or a literal punishment—she could not illustrate her point with a "clearly sane" and innocent heroine because such a woman would not be a deviant. More importantly, however, Matus assumes that Braddon would be on the side of the social deviant rather than on the side of those trying to incarcerate social deviants. This is a typical mistake for contemporary critics, who generally let their own modern sensibilities cloud their reading of the novel. Many critics have read *Lady Audley's Secret* as a subversive tale about the vulnerability of women in Victorian England and the danger women face in deviating from societal norms. Moreover, they interpret Lady Audley's institutionalization as a metaphor. In doing so, they ignore the specific cases of people wrongly institutionalized that were circulating in England during the time Braddon's story was written. Furthermore, they ignore Braddon's personal responses to these cases. When *Lady Audley's Secret* is examined in relation to the incarceration scare, it becomes clear that the dominant modern interpretation of the novel is inadequate. Braddon's most famous novel is *not* subversive. Instead of condemning the impulse to punish deviance,

Braddon actually acknowledges it as a necessary means of protecting society.

CHAPTER SEVEN

"MAKING MISCHIEF": THE DEPRESSION, TREATMENT, AND WORK OF CHARLOTTE PERKINS GILMAN

While some women of the Victorian and Modern periods were labeled mad and punished for their unconventional behavior, other women truly experienced mind and mood disorders that impaired their ability to function. One of the latter is Charlotte Perkins Gilman. In the midst of a depression in 1887, Gilman wrote a letter detailing her illness to a doctor whose rest home she was about to visit for treatment. In 1892 Gilman published "The Yellow Wallpaper," a short story inspired by her own experience with depression and the treatment she received. Towards the end of her life, Gilman also wrote an autobiography detailing the true account of her lifelong struggle with mental illness. In these texts, Gilman not only paints a vivid portrait of a woman suffering from psychological distress, she also protests how mentally ill women are treated by the medical community and the public at large.

In both the 1887 letter to her doctor and the 1935 autobiography, Gilman suggests that her mental breakdown was triggered by pregnancy. She reports experiencing "terrible fits of remorse and depression," and "'nervousness'" during her confinement (Letter 273). Moreover, it was during this time that she began having "wild and dreadful ideas which [she] was powerless to check, times of excitement and times of tears" (Letter 273). According to her autobiography, "We had attributed all my increasing weakness and depression to pregnancy" (*Living* 88-89).

It is not unusual for childbirth to trigger depression. In the nineteenth century, mental illness caused by childbirth was termed puerperal insanity. In the last decades of the century, puerperal insanity was listed as the cause of admission for at least ten percent of women in insane asylums (Theriot, "Diagnosing" 405). Symptoms included trouble sleeping, nonsensical speech, incessant weeping, and "acting generally peculiar" (Theriot, "Negotiating" 354)—all symptoms exhibited by the heroine of "The Yellow Wallpaper." In "Under the Shadow of Maternity," Judith

Walzer Leavitt explains the danger and fear surrounding childbirth in the nineteenth century. Although deaths related to childbirth were declining during the fin de siècle, they remained high (Leavitt 332). Most women knew someone who had died in childbirth, and expectant mothers worried they would not survive the delivery. Moreover, if childbirth didn't kill a woman, it could still maim her for life. In 1897 one doctor noted, "widespread mutilation . . . is so common, indeed, that we scarcely find a normal perineal after childbirth" (qtd. in Leavitt 334). In fact, the increased use of forceps in the delivery room near the end of the century led to an increased incidence of accidental perineal and cervical mutilations (Leavitt 336). One must sympathize with the woman who wrote of her 1885 delivery, "Between oceans of pain, there stretched continents of fear; fear of death and dread of suffering beyond bearing" (qtd. in Leavitt 337). The threat to bodily integrity posed by childbirth in the nineteenth century made it an extremely traumatic event, so the high incidence of insanity associated with childbirth is understandable.

On top of worrying about the threat to their own lives and limbs, mothers also had to worry about the lives of their unborn children. Charlotte Perkins Gilman was undoubtedly aware that her baby might not live through the delivery. Her oldest sibling "died from some malpractice at birth" (*Living* 8), and another sibling "died in infancy" (*Living* 11). Her grandmother lost her first baby as well (*Living* 7). After Gilman's birth, "The doctor said that if my mother had another baby she would die," prompting her father to abandon the family (*Living* 5). For Gilman, childbirth must have been associated with bereavement.

Gilman's letter and autobiography suggest that her depression developed during pregnancy. However, her spirits did not improve after the baby's birth. Indeed, in the 1887 letter to her doctor, Gilman implies that her depression deepened after childbirth: "This agony of mind set in with the child's coming. I nursed her in slow tears. All that summer I did nothing but cry, save for times when the pain was unbearable and I grew wild, hysterical, almost imbecile at times" (Letter 273). In her autobiography she writes: "Here was a charming home; a loving and devoted husband; an exquisite baby . . . and I lay on the couch and cried" (*Living* 89). Not only does Gilman cry all of the time, her thought processes are impaired. She explains, "I can't think, I can't remember, I can't grasp an idea. But I could once" (Letter 274). According to Kay Redfield Jamison, a clinical psychologist and co-director of the Mood Disorder Center at Johns Hopkins University, "[w]hen energy is profoundly dissipated, the ability to think is clearly eroded, and the capacity to actively engage in the efforts and pleasures of life is fundamentally altered, then depression becomes an illness rather than a temporary or existential state" (18). Writing of this period thirty years later, Gilman's despair is still fresh, as she laments not understanding how she came to be "a mental wreck" in "an extreme nervous exhaustion" (*Living* 89).

In addition to feeling tired and mentally foggy, helplessness and shame are two common symptoms of depression that Gilman experienced. Such feelings dominated Gilman's mind, squeezing out positive feelings. Only those who have experienced it can understand how melancholia "consists of every painful mental sensation, shame, fear, remorse, a blind oppressive confusion, utter weakness, a steady brain-ache that fills the conscious mind with crowding images of distress" (*Living* 90). Gilman continues, "one remembers every mistake and misdeeds of a lifetime, and grovels to the earth in abasement" (*Living* 91). She is so tired she can *do nothing* except cry: "I lay on that lounge and wept all day. The tears ran down into my ears on either side. I went to bed crying, woke in the night crying, sat on the edge of the bed in the morning and cried" (*Living* 91).

While dealing with depression must be difficult for anyone, the response of others certainly did not help Gilman recover. She felt ashamed at her helplessness and guilty that "the doctors examined me and found nothing the matter" (*Living* 91). Even worse was the cynical response of others to her diagnosis of nervous prostration: "there were many who openly scoffed, saying it was only a new name for laziness" (*Living* 90). Even her friends seem to doubt her, urging Gilman, "use your will" (*Living* 90). Her mother nags her: "If you would get up and do something you would feel better," but after failing in her attempt to sweep the floor, Gilman "wept again in helpless shame" (*Living* 91).

After five months of the depression, a doctor finally suggests that Gilman "go away, for a change" (*Living* 92). When she does, a miraculous yet disturbing thing happens—she feels better. If Gilman had simply recovered from her illness and remained well, she might have been diagnosed with puerperal insanity, though that usually didn't last more than a few months (Theriot, "Negotiating" 354). However, unfortunately for Gilman, her illness returned as soon as she did (*Living* 95). The resulting depression was made worse by the thought that her illness was associated with the home: "This was a worse horror than before, for now I saw the stark fact—that I was well while away and sick while at home—a heartening prospect!" (*Living* 95). Gilman's depression continued until she and her husband were sure she would go insane.

In 1887 a friend of Gilman's mother gave her the money to seek treatment in the rest home of Silas Weir Mitchell, "the first authority on nervous diseases" (Gilman, Letter 273). Before her arrival, Gilman wrote

Mitchell a long letter describing her illness. She tells him, "There is something the matter with my head. No one here knows or believes or cares" (Letter 274). She begs him "not to laugh at me as every one else does" (Letter 273). In addition to pleading for Mitchell to take her illness seriously, Gilman also apprises him of her intellectual work:

> I am a writer, a poet, a philosopher, in little. I am a teacher by instinct and profession. I am a reader and thinker. I can do some good work for the world if I live. I cannot bear to die or go insane or linger on [in] this wretched invalid existence, and be a weight on this poor world which has so many now. I want to work, to help people, to do good. I did for years, and can again if I get well. (Letter 273-74)

While Mitchell did take Gilman's illness seriously—she was promptly diagnosed with hysteria (Gilman, *Living* 95)—the same cannot be said of her work. As Ann Douglas Wood explains, "Professional work . . . was hardly a socially acceptable escape from a lady's situation, but sickness, that very nervous condition brought on by the frustrations of her life, was" (36).

From Mitchell's perspective, the intellectual work that Gilman sought to continue was the cause of her illness in the first place. Victorian physicians argued that a woman only had a limited amount of energy, and that energy was required for the development of her uterus and ovaries. According to this theory, if a woman spent her energy on masculine pursuits like education or work, she would very likely go insane. Mitchell subscribed to this theory himself, saying, "The woman's desire to be on a level of competition with men and to assume his duties is, I am sure, making mischief" (*Doctor* 13). The proper treatment for a woman whose illness is caused by her attempts to step outside of woman's role and into man's involves reinforcing the ideology of separate spheres. Ann Douglas Wood explains: "Since her disease was unconsciously viewed as a symptom of a failure in femininity, its remedy was designed both as a punishment and an agent of regeneration, for it forced her to acknowledge her womanhood" (37). Thus, "nervous women were advised to recognize their biological limitations and devote themselves exclusively to domesticity and the home" (Bederman 130). In addition to discouraging masculine pursuits and encouraging domesticity, physicians who practiced the "rest cure" required their female patients to surrender control and assume a role of complete dependence, a role that was associated with women in nineteenth-century culture.

In *Fat and Blood*, Mitchell explains that his "rest cure" involves keeping the patient in bed for six to eight weeks. During much of this time, he does "not permit the patient to sit up, or to sew or write or read, or to use the hands in any active way except to clean the teeth" (Mitchell, *Fat* 58). This means that feeding, bathing, and "all correspondence [is] carried on through the nurse" (Mitchell, *Fat* 60). In the early stages of treatment, Weir Mitchell doesn't even allow patients to get up to relieve themselves, but "arrange[s] to have the bowels and water passed while lying down" (Mitchell, *Fat* 59). In addition to forcing a state of dependency on the patient, the doctor must "teach the sick person how very essential it is to speak of her aches and pains to no one but himself" (Mitchell, *Fat* 62). By infantilizing the patient, the "rest cure" reinforces the passive, weak, dependent, silent role a woman is supposed to play in nineteenth-century culture.

Gilman seems to have responded well to being under Mitchell's care, as did many other women. However, she did not fare so well after Mitchell released her with directions to "Live as domestic a life as possible. Have your child with you all the time. . . . Have but two hours' intellectual life a day. And never touch pen, brush, or pencil as long as you live'" (*Living* 96). When Gilman "followed those directions rigidly for months," she "came perilously near to losing [her] mind" (*Living* 96). Though she evidently did not rip up the wallpaper, she "would crawl into remote closets and under beds—to hide from the grinding pressure of that profound distress" (*Living* 96).

While Mitchell treated Gilman by trying to force her back into the domestic sphere, "Gilman realized that for her the traditional domestic role was at least in part the cause of her distress" (Treichler 68). She accepted the medical theory that she only had a limited amount of energy, but she thought that *she* should determine how that energy be spent. Gilman wrote: "We have a certain storage of nerve force, with which we can drive ourselves. . . . For the conscious mind to compel the body to do what it has no inherited desire or acquired habit of doing, is a direct expense" (qtd. in Thrailkill 541). In an article on "The 'Nervous Breakdown' of Women," Gilman elaborates:

> Full nervous serenity depends on the smooth adjustment of the two interacting parts of every living thing—the body and the spirit. The creature must be satisfied with itself; it must do what it likes to do, and like to do what it does. Any caged animal shows the effect on the nervous system of interference with natural physical habits. (203)

For Gilman, life in the domestic sphere was akin to life in a cage. While Victorian physicians believed that women might lose their minds if they stepped outside of their proper gender role, Gilman thought that enforcing gender roles may actually be the root of the problem. Thus, the doctors who enforced cultural notions of gender and prohibited women from work outside of the domestic sphere were actually exacerbating mental illness in some women. For her, domestic work was what was "making mischief," not intellectual work.

In 1888—two and a half years after the birth of their daughter—Gilman and her husband decided to separate. Gilman believed that the role of wife—not just the role of mother—caused her illness and a separation would return her to health: "This miserable condition of mind, this darkness, feebleness and gloom, had begun in those difficult years of courtship, had grown rapidly worse after marriage, and was now threatening utter loss; whereas I had repeated proof that the moment I left home I began to recover. It seemed right to give up a mistaken marriage" (*Living* 97). However, for the rest of her life Gilman continued to battle depression. Gilman persists in blaming the marriage for her mental illness: "If this decision could have been reached sooner it would have been much better for me, the lasting mental injury would have been less. Such recovery as I have made in forty years, and the work accomplished, seem to show that the fear of insanity was not fulfilled, but the effects of nerve bankruptcy remain to this day" (*Living* 97). However, Gilman's health is not as steadily poor as "nerve bankruptcy" might suggest. Though she continued to experience periods of depression, Gilman also experienced periods when she was high-functioning, which she considered to be normal.

The diary entries that Gilman includes in her autobiography indicate that this depressive episode persists for at least a few years after the separation. She variously records feelings of lethargy, hopelessness, self-blame, and guilt, as well as slowed thinking, impaired concentration, and thoughts of death, all of which are signs of depression (Jamison 13). Moreover, she tells us, "There were plenty of blanks in this diary. . . . The blanks were the drowned time, not even sense to make those scanty notes" (*Living* 115). While she was evidently very depressed, Gilman was functioning enough to support herself, her daughter, and her mother. By this time her mother was more taxing than her child. A winter diary entry for 1891 reads: "Dr. Kellog in. She doubts if I can stand the strain of our present family arrangement much longer" (*Living* 135). Gilman explains that "The 'strain' was with mother" (*Living* 135). While she trudges on, Gilman's diary entries continue to be as bleak as they were before the separation. In one entry she writes of "the black helplessness into which I fell, with its deadness of heart, its aching emptiness of mind," and how her daughter would "bring me a handkerchief because she saw my tears" (*Living* 154).

While Gilman's depression lasts for several years, her moods start to gradually fluctuate. In 1893, her mother dies and her ex-husband remarries her best friend. She does not mention her feelings upon her mother's death, but she is reportedly pleased with the marriage: "My sense of gladness, of relief, that some happiness could have been established after so much unhappiness, was intense" (*Living* 167). After the marriage, Gilman arranges to send her daughter to the east coast to live with her father. In 1895 Gilman begins a nomadic life, roaming the country giving lectures and writing articles. Although Gilman still comments frequently on her periods of depression, bursts of feverish energy interrupt such low periods. To Gilman, these periods of intense activity are just interludes of normalcy.[1] Gilman brags that she wrote *Women and Economics* "in seventeen days, in five different houses, on this little string of visits" (*Living* 237). For seven years Gilman ran the *Forerunner*, a monthly magazine, completely on her own. Each issue had an installment of a novel, an installment of a book, a short story, articles, poems, verses, allegories, humor, and book reviews (*Living* 305). Her bibliographer lists 2,168 published works (See Scharnhorst).

Because of her phenomenal productivity, Gilman's friends fail to notice her bouts of melancholia. She frequently complains that people do not understand how severe her depressions are, that they do not believe that she suffers because she is always so industrious. She writes, "since my public activities do not show weakness, nor my writings, and since brain and nerve disorder is not visible, short of lunacy or general 'prostration,' this lifetime of limitation and wretchedness, when I mention it, is flatly disbelieved" (*Living* 98). While we see evidence of depressive episodes repeatedly in her diary entries, her friends have not had this perspective. Indeed, it seems as though her reason for publishing the autobiography is to prove to her friends how ill she has been. She writes, "friends gibber amiably, 'I wish I had your mind!' I wish they had, for a while, as punishment for doubting my word. What confuses them is the visible work I have been able to accomplish. They say activity, achievement, they do not see blank months of idleness" (*Living* 98). She complains, "the humiliating loss of a large part of one's brain power, of more than half one's working life, accompanied with deep misery and anguish of mind—this when complained of is met with amiable laughter and flat disbelief" (*Living* 104). Gilman believes that her "output of work could have almost been trebled" if she didn't have low points of "extreme distress, shame, discouragement, misery. Is a loss like this, suffering like this, to be met with light laughter

[1] Such periods of astounding activity may be indicative of mania. According to Kay Redfield Jamison, artists tend to interpret episodes of mania as "creative inspiration" and a normal part of their personality (58).

and compliments?" (*Living* 103). Though her extensive body of work and her unbelievably-full schedule of lectures made it difficult for friends to recognize her illness, Gilman's work is also what allowed her to overcome her periods of depression.

According to Gilman, she recovered through "work, the normal life of every human being; work, in which is joy and growth and service, without which one is a pauper and a parasite" ("Why"). In recovering from her worst depressive episode, Gilman's work included "The Yellow Wallpaper." Gilman described "The Yellow Wallpaper" as "a case of nervous breakdown beginning something as mine did, and treated as Dr. S. Weir Mitchell treated me with what I consider to be the inevitable result, insanity" (*Living* 119). Gilman said "that she didn't consider the work to be 'literature' at all, that everything she wrote was for a purpose, in this case that of pointing out the dangers of a particular medical treatment" (Shumaker 589). Gilman wrote "The Yellow Wallpaper" in an effort "to work, to help people, to do good" (Letter 274)—an activity that was prohibited by the very treatment she critiques.

Gilman used her own experience with mental illness and its treatment as inspiration in writing "The Yellow Wallpaper." The narrator's inability to enjoy her baby implies that her depression was triggered by its birth: "Such a dear baby! And yet I *cannot* be with him, it makes me so nervous" ("Yellow" 6). And like Gilman, her heroine shows signs of depression. The narrator laments: "I cry at nothing, and cry most of the time" ("Yellow" 9). Moreover, the narrator of the story is also tired all the time ("Yellow" 10). In addition to these symptoms, the narrator says, "It is getting to be a great effort for me to think straight" ("Yellow" 11). Crying, fatigue, and impaired mental function are all symptoms of depression that Gilman experienced herself and passed on to the narrator of "The Yellow Wallpaper."

In addition to describing the symptoms of depression in "The Yellow Wallpaper," Gilman reveals how damaging other people's reactions to depression can be. The narrator's husband scoffs at her: "John does not know how much I really suffer. He knows there is no *reason* to suffer, and that satisfies him" (6). John assures his wife that she is not really ill: "You see he does not believe I am sick!" ("Yellow" 3). When she tries to talk to him about her illness, John says: "Bless her little heart! . . . she shall be as sick as she pleases!" ("Yellow" 12). His belittling attitude towards his wife shames and frustrates her, feelings that are all the more magnified by his supposed authority. He is a doctor whose "serious cases" are in contrast to that of his wife ("Yellow" 6). She asks: "If a physician of high standing, and one's own husband, assures friends and relatives that there is really nothing the matter . . . what is one to do?" ("Yellow" 3-4). As the story plays out, it is clear that her husband doesn't want her "to do" anything. She has very little agency over her own life or the treatment that she receives for her depression.

The narrator's course of treatment in "The Yellow Wallpaper" is modeled after the "rest cure" that Gilman received at the hands of Silas Weir Mitchell. In comparison to the treatment Mitchell describes in his books, the "rest cure" imposed on the narrator of the "The Yellow Wallpaper" is relatively mild. Indeed, the story itself suggests that Mitchell's treatment is more extreme. The narrator writes: "John says if I don't pick up faster he shall send me to Weir Mitchell in the fall. But I don't want to go there at all. I had a friend who was in his hands once, and she says he is just like John and my brother, only more so!" ("Yellow" 9).

The lack of control patients of the "rest cure" had is mimicked in "The Yellow Wallpaper, where Gilman highlights how infantilizing such treatment is. The narrator's husband forces her to stay in the nursery, carries her to bed, and calls her "little girl" ("Yellow" 12). She says he "hardly lets me stir without special direction" ("Yellow" 5). As Gilman's story brilliantly illustrates, this treatment infantilizes the patient, making her completely helpless and dependent on others. This lack of control is literally maddening, though it is billed as a benevolent treatment. The narrator explains: "he takes all care from me, and I feel basely ungrateful not to value it more" ("Yellow" 5). Not only does the lack of agency make the narrator feel like a child, it makes her feel like a prisoner. The windows of her room are barred, there are chains in the walls, a gate is at the top of the stairs, and the bed is nailed to the floor. The woman trapped behind bars in the pattern of the wallpaper is obviously a reflection of the narrator herself ("Yellow" 16).

While Charlotte Perkins Gilman was forced to take a passive, silent role as a patient of the "rest cure," she seized an active, vocal role when she wrote about her experience with this treatment in "The Yellow Wallpaper." In writing this short story, Gilman's stated purpose was "to save people from being driven crazy" by exposing the disastrous results that this type of treatment could have on a patient ("Why"). According to Gilman, she succeeded in accomplishing this: "It has, to my knowledge, saved one woman from a similar fate—so terrifying her family that they let her out into normal activity and she recovered" ("Why"). Gilman also claims that Mitchell "had altered his treatment of neurasthenia since reading *The Yellow Wallpaper*" ("Why"), though Mitchell's publications do not reflect this (Dock et al. 62).

According to Gilman, the "rest cure" did not lead to her recovery. However, she gradually wandered down the path towards recovery without medical advice. It may have been impossible for Gilman to heal without reconstructing her own story (see Herman). The most well-known way to do this is through talk therapy, but Gilman was critical of the craze for "Freudian psychology" in New York: "Always it amazed me to see how apparently intelligent persons would permit these mind-meddlers, having no claim to fitness except that of having read utterly unproven books, to paddle among their thoughts and feelings, and extract confessions of the last intimacy" (*Living* 314). When she refused one analyst's pleas that she "come to be 'psyched,'" he "had the impudence to write a long psychoanalysis of my case, and send it to me" (*Living* 314). Gilman promptly ordered her husband to burn it without reading it. One must, indeed, wonder how therapeutic that psychoanalyst would have been if he thought he could do all the talking himself.

Though Gilman did not want to talk through her feelings herself, it is interesting to note that the narrator in "The Yellow Wallpaper" does. She explains, "It is so hard to talk with John about my case" ("Yellow" 12). She repeatedly mentions how she *wants* to talk about her condition and her feelings with her husband, but—like Mitchell—he discourages her from complaining. On one occasion when she "thought it was a good time to talk" about changing her supposed treatment, John interrupts her, saying: "you really are better, dear, whether you see it or not. I am a doctor, dear, and I know" ("Yellow" 12). When she again tries to voice her own feelings about her mental state, he "looked at me with such a stern, reproachful look that I could not say another word" ("Yellow" 13). John discourages his wife from voicing her feelings, "so of course I said no more on that score" ("Yellow" 13). Perhaps unconsciously, the story suggests the dangers of denying the patient the ability to talk about her feelings.

Gilman was evidently reluctant to voice her narrative herself, but she was eventually able to write it. Writing her narrative was an act of scriptotherapy. As Suzette Henke explains, scriptotherapy is "the process of writing out and writing through traumatic experience in the mode of therapeutic reenactment" (xii). As Henke has suggested, life-writing can be "a therapeutic alternative" to the talking cure "for victims of severe anxiety and, more seriously, of post-traumatic stress disorder" (xiii). Henke explains, "the life-writing project generates a healing narrative that temporarily restores the fragmented self to an empowered position of psychological agency" (xvi). Gilman made progress towards this end early in her illness by writing "The Yellow Wallpaper." Not only was this text an act of scriptotherapy, it actually advocates scriptotherapy. The story's narrator expresses the belief that writing can be therapeutic: "I think sometimes that if I were only able to write a little it would relieve the press of ideas and rest me" ("Yellow" 7). Like Gilman, the narrator decides to write her story because she cannot speak it: "I don't know why I should write this. . . . But I *must* say what I feel and think in some way—it is such a relief!" ("Yellow" 10).

While writing "The Yellow Wallpaper" must have been therapeutic for Gilman, this work of fiction does not fully explore the psychological roots of her depression. And although Gilman had kept diaries for years, these were largely unhelpful. According to Judith Herman, a professor of clinical psychiatry at Harvard Medical School, "[t]he recitation of facts without the accompanying emotions is a sterile exercise, without therapeutic effect" (177). In her autobiography, Gilman mentions that her "purpose in diary-keeping, since girlhood, was not at all to make revelations of feeling, thoughts" (*Living* 244).

One must wonder if Gilman continued to suffer from depressive episodes after she wrote her autobiography. Although the last chapter is written ten years after the rest of the book, she makes no mention of mental illness. Though Gilman may have finally escaped the mental illness that plagued most of her life, she was not allowed to enjoy recovery long. In 1932 she discovered she had breast cancer, and she "utterly refused a late operation," though she did try "X-ray treatment" (*Living* 334). The woman whose doctor deprived her of autonomy was not going to let this final decision be made for her. She writes, "I had not the least objection to dying. But I did not propose to die of this, so I promptly bought sufficient chloroform as a substitute" (*Living* 333). Gilman ended her own life on August 17th, 1935, shortly after completing her autobiography. Just as she refused to play the role of passive female during her life, she consciously chose to play an active role in her own death. In doing so, she rejected the treatment prescribed for cancer just as she had rejected the treatment prescribed for hysteria. Moreover, she continued to make mischief until the very end by criticizing both treatments in her work.

CHAPTER EIGHT

MADNESS AND MAD DOCTORS IN THE LIFE AND WORK OF VIRGINIA WOOLF

Like Charlotte Perkins Gilman, Virginia Woolf suffered from mental illness for most of her life. And like Gilman, Woolf not only incorporated her experiences with mental illness into her work, she used that work to critique the doctors who treated her. Woolf's illness was likely triggered by the traumas she experienced in the developmental stages of her life. When Woolf was thirteen years old, her mother died. Her sister Stella took over the role of nurturing maternal figure, only to die two years later. The deaths of these two central figures left psychological scars on Woolf that would never heal. The death of her father when she was just eighteen was another blow to Woolf, as was the death of her brother Thoby when she was twenty-four. In addition to the deaths in her family, Woolf had to cope with the sexual abuse she suffered at the hands of her half-brothers George and Gerald Duckworth. The tragedies in her life were undoubtedly related to the periods of psychological distress that Woolf suffered from since the death of her mother in 1895 until her own death in 1941.

Woolf's experience with mental illness was traumatic in and of itself. She heard voices, had recurrent bouts of depression, suffered from delusions, and had disabling migraines. Despite all of these symptoms, Woolf often said there was nothing truly wrong with her and blamed herself for her own emotional problems and for the problems of those around her. During her depressive moods, Woolf sometimes felt as though she deserved to be punished, and she often refused to eat. Over the course of her life, she had several breakdowns in which she went "mad" and was institutionalized, and she attempted suicide twice unsuccessfully. While these bouts of mental illness would have been traumatic for anyone, they must have been especially disturbing to Woolf, as the permanent institutionalization of her half-sister Laura Stephen loomed over her as an ever-present threat of her own possible fate.

Woolf visited a rest home four different times over the course of her life, in addition to being treated by several eminent physicians. However, as Stephen Trombley explains: "None of them were much help, and some even made her situation more difficult" (9). Based on her own writings, it would certainly seem as though Woolf did not think highly of her doctors or their proffered treatments. Woolf wrote: "My life is a constant fight against Doctors follies, it seems to me" (*Letters* 1: 163). While some of her symptoms might have been alleviated if she had been able to talk through the traumas she had experienced, she did not experience that form of treatment. Her brother Adrian and his wife were both doctors who were trained in psychoanalysis under Freud, and she and her husband Leonard published English translations of Freud's collected works through the Hogarth Press. However, Woolf—like Charlotte Perkins Gilman—was skeptical of the talking cure. She wrote to a friend: "We could all go on like that for hours; and yet these Germans think it proves something—besides their own gull-like imbecility" (*Letters* 3: 135).

While Woolf never tried talk therapy, writing about the tragedies in her life may have been therapeutic. As Suzette Henke explains: "Autobiography could so effectively mimic the scene of psychoanalysis that life-writing might provide a therapeutic alternative" (xiii). Writing about traumatic experiences in an effort to develop a meaningful and coherent narrative about them could serve as a form of catharsis. Thus, Woolf's diary entries, letters, and autobiographical essays may have helped to alleviate her psychological wounds. However, Woolf's novels may also be examined as examples of scriptotherapy, for many of them allude to the tragic circumstances that scarred her.

To the Lighthouse is the novel that most obviously addresses the personal loss Woolf felt upon the death of a loved one. Not only does this novel recreate both of Woolf's parents in the characters of Mr. and Mrs. Ramsay, it explores the death of her mother and the effect it had on the rest of her family. Moreover, the novel touches on the deaths of Stella and Thoby as well. Like Stella's, Prue's death is a result of "some illness connected to childbirth" (*TTL* 135). And although Thoby did not die in combat like Andrew, to Woolf both deaths represent the waste of young life. Writing *To the Lighthouse* was an exercise in scriptotherapy for Woolf, as she herself suggests: "I expressed some very long felt and deeply felt emotion. And in expressing it I explained it and then laid it to rest" (Woolf *MOB* 81).

Though writing *To the Lighthouse* might have given Woolf some sense of closure, it was neither the first nor the last time that she would allude to the losses of her loved ones in fictional form. Like Woolf, both Clarissa of *Mrs. Dalloway* and Rachel Vinrace of *The Voyage Out* have lost their mothers at an early age. The death of Mrs. Pargiter in *The Years* bears a more obvious resemblance to the death of Julia Stephen, as she too left behind a grieving husband and a house full of children. While Thoby Stephen's death is alluded to in *To the Lighthouse*, it is explored more fully through the deaths of the title character of *Jacob's Room* and Percival in *The Waves*. The death of her sister Sylvia is also traumatic for Clarissa Dalloway, just as Stella's death was to Woolf.

In addition to addressing the effects of the death of a loved one, Woolf's novels reference other traumatic experiences in her life. Both Rhoda in *The Waves* and Septimus in *Mrs. Dalloway* commit suicide; indeed, Septimus kills himself by jumping out a window, as Woolf tried to do after the death of her father. The trauma inflicted by sexual abuse is also alluded to in some of her novels, though it is not explicit. In *The Years*, ten-year old Rose must cope with a traumatic encounter in which a man exposes himself to her on the street, and Helen "suspected [Rachel's father] of nameless atrocities with regard to his daughter" in *The Voyage Out* (24). Furthermore, Rachel's nightmare reflects Woolf's own history of childhood sexual abuse:

> She dreamt that she was walking down a long tunnel, which grew so narrow by degrees that she could touch the damp bricks on either side. At length the tunnel opened and became a vault; she found herself trapped in it, bricks meeting her wherever she turned, alone with a little deformed man who squatted on the floor gibbering, with long nails. His face was pitted and like the face of an animal. The wall behind him oozed with damp, which collected into drops and slid down. (77)

Patricia Cramer argues that "Woolf specifically revisits the scene of George Duckworth's sexual violation" in this nightmare (19). Woolf's history of sexual abuse would certainly explain such a nightmare, though perhaps the abuse she suffered at the hands of Gerald Duckworth is more relevant here. In "A Sketch of the Past," Woolf associates her sexual abuse at the hands of Gerald with an incident when she was frightened when looking in the mirror: "I dreamt that I was looking in a glass when a horrible face—the face of an animal—suddenly showed over my shoulder" (*MOB* 69). In the nightmares of both Woolf and Rachel, this "face of an animal" replaces the face of the abuser. Moreover, the "long nails" of the man inside the tunnels of Rachel's dream could very well symbolize the nails of Gerald, whose "hand explored [Woolf's] private parts" (*MOB* 69). For Rachel, Richard Dalloway's kiss is an act of sexual aggression which triggers this nightmare about male penetration.

While Woolf explores the traumas of her life to varying degrees in several novels, the novel that most reflects her experience with mental illness is *Mrs. Dalloway.* Through the voices of Clarissa and Septimus, Woolf leaves behind her own lyrical description of her illness. Rather than burdening one character with all of her psychological baggage, Woolf created two characters that experience psychological distress on two distinctly different levels. Septimus is in a state of constant flux between moments of depression and moments of manic delusion. Clarissa, on the other hand, exhibits none of the delusions symptomatic of mania, though she has recurrent moments of depression.

Although Clarissa's moments of psychological distress are triggered by criticism, the ultimate root of her depression is trauma. Peter explains how Clarissa's outlook on life was shaped by the death of her sister:

> Those ruffians, the Gods, shan't have it all their own way,—her notion being that the Gods, who never lost a chance in hurting, thwarting and spoiling human lives were seriously put out if, all the same, you behaved like a lady. That phase came directly after Sylvia's death—that horrible affair. To see your own sister killed by a falling tree (all Justin Parry's fault—all his carelessness) before your very eyes, a girl too on the verge of life, the most gifted of them, Clarissa always said, was enough to turn one bitter. (*MD* 76)

The death of her sister does more than inspire bitterness—it causes a change in Clarissa's existential outlook and has probably contributed to her periods of depression.

Throughout her life, Woolf experienced bouts of depression, and those experiences are reflected in the melancholy moods of Clarissa in *Mrs. Dalloway*. Clarissa's thoughts reveal how quickly depression can attack:

> But-but-why did she suddenly feel, for no reason that she could discover, desperately unhappy? . . . It was a feeling, some unpleasant feeling, earlier in the day perhaps; something that Peter had said, combined with some depression of her own, in her bedroom, taking off her hat; and what Richard had said had added to it, but what had he said? There were his roses. Her parties! That was it! Her parties! Both of them criticized her very unfairly, laughed at her unjustly, for her parties. That was it! That was it! (*MD* 117-18)

The key to triggering Clarissa's bouts of depression, as well as Woolf's, is public scrutiny. Woolf put herself under constant pressure to gain society's approval. Consequently, every literary publication was a matter of extreme importance because Woolf used its success or failure to determine her own position in society, much as Mrs. Dalloway uses her parties to gauge society's opinion of her.

Both Clarissa Dalloway and Virginia Woolf are aware that their bouts of depression coincide with times when they feel most vulnerable to criticism. After the publication of *The Voyage Out*, Woolf and those closest to her were able to locate the immediate source of her breakdown. Her sister Vanessa wrote to a friend "Please be very careful not to say a word to anyone about her worrying over what people will think of her novel, which seems really to be the entire cause of her breakdown" (qtd. in Bell 2: 12). Similarly, Clarissa recognizes that her parties trigger moments of psychological distress: "Oh, dear, it was going to be a failure; a complete failure, Clarissa felt it in her bones… She could see Peter out of the tail of her eye, criticizing her, there, in the corner. Why, after all, did she do these things? Why seek pinnacles and stand drenched in fire?" (*MD* 163). Clarissa seeks to achieve pinnacles of success through parties the same way that Woolf seeks to achieve them through books, but by attempting to gain society's approval both women place themselves under scrutiny. In turn, this scrutiny spawns their depressions.

When Clarissa feels herself to be under the extreme pressure precipitated by such scrutiny, she becomes panicked:

> Then (she had felt it only this morning) there was the terror; the overwhelming incapacity, one's parents giving it into one's hands, this life, to be lived to the end, to be walked with serenely; there was in the depths of her heart an awful fear. Even now, quite often if Richard had not been there reading the *Times*, so that she could crouch like a bird and gradually revive, send roaring up that immeasurable delight, rubbing stick to stick, one thing with another, she must have perished. (*MD* 180)

In this description, Clarissa reveals the anxiety she feels during acute stages of depression, and she implies that the only reason she has not "perished" is because of Richard's presence, which allows her to "gradually revive." In her suicide letter, Woolf expresses a similar reliance on her husband, telling him "If anyone could have saved me it would have been you" (qtd. in Bell 2: 226). Although Clarissa suffers from a mental illness modeled after Woolf's personal experience, her ability to withstand the depressive phases, as well as the absence of manic symptoms, indicates that Woolf bequeathed to

Clarissa a much milder form of mental illness than she bestowed on Septimus.[1]

When reading *Mrs. Dalloway*, it becomes obvious to the reader that Septimus Smith is mentally ill and that his mental illness was triggered by the trauma of war. Like Woolf, Septimus ultimately ends his own life because he is unable to cope with his illness. Although both Woolf and Septimus sought medical assistance, neither received the kind of treatment that could offer the hope of recovery. By recreating her own experiences of mental illness through Septimus, Woolf attempted to heal herself through scriptotherapy and indict the medical practices that harmed rather than healed her.

Although there are many signs that Septimus suffers from trauma, he is perhaps most troubled by symptoms of constriction. Septimus displays symptoms of anhedonia—the inability to feel—immediately upon Evans's death: "when Evans was killed, just before the Armistice, in Italy, Septimus, far from showing any emotion or recognizing that here was the end of a friendship, congratulated himself upon feeling very little and very reasonably. The War had taught him. . . . The last shells had missed him. He watched them explode with indifference" (*MD* 84). Septimus initially congratulates himself for his inability to feel, as this numbness helps him to cope with war. However, he realizes that the continuance of these feelings after the war is unhealthy: "For now that it was all over, truce signed, and the dead buried, he had, especially in the evening, these sudden thunderclaps of fear. He could not feel. . . . he could not feel" (*MD* 85). Septimus's anhedonia not only prevents him from feeling pain; it prevents him from feeling pleasure: "But beauty was behind a pane of glass. Even taste . . . had no relish to him. . . . But he could not taste, he could not feel. In the teashop among the tables and the waiters the appalling fear came over him that he could not feel" (*MD* 86). Septimus's anhedonia sends him into a panic: "he became engaged one evening when the panic was on him—that he could not feel" (*MD* 85).

In "A Sketch of the Past," Woolf describes a similar numbness at her mother's deathbed: "I remember very clearly how even as I was taken to the bedside I noticed that one nurse was sobbing, and a desire to laugh came over me, and I said to myself as I have often done at moments of crisis since, 'I feel nothing whatever'" (*MOB* 92). To deal with her mother's death, Woolf's body went into shock, making it impossible for her to feel

[1] In the 1928 introduction to *Mrs. Dalloway*, Woolf claimed that she originally planned to have Clarissa commit suicide, but she created Septimus to die in her place (Scott xlviii).

pain. Woolf recreated her own experience with trauma through Septimus, a character whose defense against pain is to become numb to it.

Septimus desperately struggles to understand the cause of his anhedonia: "He could reason; he could read . . . his brain was perfect; it must be the fault of the world then—that he could not feel" (*MD* 86). Septimus comes to fear that "it might be possible that the world itself is without meaning" (*MD* 86). As Karen DeMeester explains, "Though Septimus's anhedonia or inability to feel begins before the end of the war, it is perpetuated and exacerbated by his inability to find meaning either in his war experiences or in his suffering during and after those experiences" (82). Traumatic events "violate the victim's faith in a natural or divine order and cast the victim into a state of existential crisis" (Herman 50). For this reason, there is "the need for survivors to give meaning to their suffering in order to recover" (DeMeester 77). Because Septimus cannot give meaning to his misery, he completely detaches himself from the world of senseless suffering: "His wife was crying, and he felt nothing; only each time she sobbed in this profound, this silent, this hopeless way, he descended another step into the pit" (*MD* 88).

Septimus's constrictive retreat from the world is a forewarning of surrender. As Kay Redfield Jamison explains, anhedonia often leads to surrender in victims of depression: "A deep sense of futility is accompanied, if not preceded, by the belief that the ability to experience pleasure is permanently gone" (18). Unable to feel pleasure or pain, the victim feels helpless. "When a person is completely powerless, and any form of resistance is futile, she may go into a state of surrender" (Herman 42). Septimus's anhedonia eventually leads him to admit defeat: "At last, with a melodramatic gesture which he assumed mechanically and with complete consciousness of its insincerity, he dropped his head in his hands. Now he had surrendered; now other people must be sent for. He gave in" (*MD* 88). After surrendering to his depression, "Nothing could rouse him" (*MD* 88). In his depression, Septimus can do nothing but lie in bed (*MD* 90). He is too weak to follow through on his suicidal ideation: "He was too weak; he could scarcely raise his hand" (*MD* 90).[2]

In addition to suffering from constriction and depression, Septimus also suffers from hyperarousal. One of the three categories of symptoms that trauma victims exhibit, hyperarousal "reflects the persistent expectation of danger" (Herman 35). The continual stress experienced during war warps the nervous system so that the victim of war trauma continues to experience

---

[2] Septimus's catatonic behavior during this period is akin to the periods of "helpless stupor" that William Styron describes in his memoir about depression (17).

the stress of battle even after leaving that environment. Victims suffer from both general anxiety and specific fears related to the traumatic event, and stimuli associated with trauma can cause the victim to relive the trauma with all of its original force. When a car backfires, Septimus is again confronted with the trauma of war, "as if some horror had come almost to the surface and was about to burst into flames" (*MD* 15). The backfire of the car, reminiscent of gunfire, triggers his memories of the war. Unable to face these memories, Septimus is "terrified" when they threaten to resurface (*MD* 15).

Septimus has all of the classic symptoms of hyperarousal: exaggerated startle reactions, irritability, psychosomatic complaints, and trouble sleeping. Practically every time Lucrezia speaks to Septimus he "started violently" (*MD* 22). One occasion when he shows both an exaggerated startle reaction and irritability is when Lucrezia prompts Septimus to "come on" and he "jumped, started, and said 'All right!' angrily, as if she had interrupted him" (*MD* 15). In addition to exaggerated startle response and irritability, Septimus suffers from "headaches, sleeplessness, fears, dreams" (*MD* 89). While victims of trauma suffer from all of these symptoms, headaches and sleeplessness are also symptoms of depression. In fact, "[d]isrupted and fitful sleep, or sleeping far too much or far too little, are among the most pervasive and consistent symptoms of depression" (Jamison 26). Although we have no indication of what Septimus's dreams are about, they may be signs of intrusion. Septimus's "dreams" could be nightmares in which he relives the traumas of war. As Judith Herman explains, intrusive symptoms occur when the traumatic moment "breaks spontaneously into consciousness, both as flashbacks during waking states and as traumatic nightmares during sleep" (37).

While Septimus clearly suffers from constriction, hyperarousal, depression, and intrusion—all classic symptoms of trauma—he also suffers from other symptoms that are not directly linked to trauma. He has paranoid, religious, and megalomaniacal delusions, all of which are common in extreme manic episodes (Herman 29). Moreover, he attaches "meanings to words of a symbolical kind" (*MD* 93). Like Woolf, Septimus appears to be suffering from mania that has been triggered by his traumatic experiences.

Many of Septimus's hallucinations feature Evans, his friend who died in battle. In one hallucination, "There was his hand; there the dead. White things were assembling behind the railings opposite. But he dared not look. Evans was behind the railings!" (*MD* 24). In another hallucination, Septimus cries: "For God's sake don't come!" because "he could not look upon the dead" (*MD* 68). At one point Evans speaks to Septimus: "Evans was speaking. The dead were with him" (*MD* 91). Speaking to the dead is another feature of Septimus's illness that is derived from Woolf's personal experiences. Just before *The Voyage Out* was released in 1915, Woolf became ill again and one morning she "began to talk to her mother" (Bell 2: 24). Of course, her mother had been dead for twenty years at this point. In many subsequent episodes of mania Woolf would continue to hear voices, and she makes this a central aspect of Septimus's hallucinations.

Speaking to the dead was just one of many ways in which Woolf's madness manifested itself. According to her nephew, "Material things assumed sinister and unpredictable aspects, beastly and terrifying or—sometimes—of fearful beauty" (Bell 2: 15). Septimus shares these hallucinations in which common objects undergo "beastly and terrifying" transformations. An example in *Mrs. Dalloway* occurs when a dog seems to transform itself into a man: "a Skye terrier snuffed his trousers and he started in an agony of fear. It was turning into a man! He could not watch it happen! It was horrible, terrible to see a dog turn into a man!" (63). While this is the most shocking example of common objects undergoing a horrific transformation in *Mrs. Dalloway*, "The Prime Minister" features similar metamorphoses.[3] In one instance, Septimus witnesses a vase spring to life: "The silver vase, with the leopard's head holding a ring in its mouth, had, too, an extreme significance, <for the leopard had opened its mouth, Septimus thought; and winked, and that had made him laugh>" (*PM* 584). This horrifying distortion of reality continues, as he attempts to "dam the hole in the wall which Septimus had made by his laugh: for something warm and disquieting had trickled through hole, and dancing over outlines of things, {making them quiver,} like hot air when it quivers over bricks" (*PM* 585). Woolf subtly hints at similar experiences in her diary: "I've had some curious visions in this room too, lying in bed, mad, & seeing the sunlight quivering like gold water, on the wall" (*Diary* 2: 283). Through the character of Septimus Smith, Woolf is able to unleash the demons that plague her, as the hallucinations he suffers are based on Woolf's own hallucinations.

Hallucinating is one of the many symptoms of extreme mania that both Woolf and Septimus exhibited. According to Jamison: "In its extreme forms mania is characterized by violent agitation, bizarre behavior, delusional thinking, and visual and auditory hallucinations" (13). Many of Septimus's hallucinations are both auditory and visual. In one instance,

[3] "The Prime Minister is the first-draft version of the opening pages of *Mrs. Dalloway*. The manuscript is located in the Berg collection of the New York Public Library, and it has been published in Bonnie Kime Scott's *Gender in Modernism*.

> He lay on the sofa and made her hold his hand to prevent him from falling down, down, he cried, into the flames! And saw faces laughing at him, calling him horrible disgusting names, from the walls, and hands pointing round the screen. Yet they were quite alone. But he began to talk aloud, answering people, arguing, laughing, crying, getting very excited and making her write things down. Perfect nonsense it was. (*MD* 65)

Flames are a recurrent visual hallucination, sometimes accompanied by screeching seagulls: "Then there were the visions. He was drowned, he used to say, and lying on a cliff with the gulls screaming over him. . . . And he would lie listening until suddenly he would cry that he was falling down, down into the flames!" (*MD* 137).

Septimus is sometimes able to recognize the reality behind his hallucinations. In one instance, "Music began clanging from the rocks up here. It is a motor horn down in the street, he muttered . . . but up here it cannoned from rock to rock . . . and became an anthem, an anthem twined round now by a shepherd boy's piping (That's an old man playing a penny whistle by the public house, he muttered)" (*MD* 67). Another hallucination is triggered when Rezia enters and "put[s] the roses in a vase, upon which the sun struck directly, and it went laughing, leaping around the room" (*MD* 91). Septimus tries to reconcile his vision of Evans with the real world where Rezia has just bought flowers from a man: "So there was a man outside; Evans presumably; and the roses, which Rezia said were half dead, had been picked by him in the fields of Greece" (*MD* 91). Septimus's ability to weave the reality of the present into his hallucinations is symptomatic of severe mania.

Septimus also suffers from paranoid delusions, which can manifest during severe episodes of mania. "He said people were talking behind the bedroom walls" (*MD* 65), and he imagined that he was "being looked at and pointed at" in the streets (*MD* 15).[4] According to Rezia, Septimus would "explain how wicked people were; how he could see them making up lies as they passed in the street. He knew all their thoughts, he said; he knew everything" (*MD* 65). Septimus lives in a delusional world where he receives messages from a higher power. When Lucrezia points out the airplane's advertisement in the sky, Septimus thinks it is a message meant for him: "So, thought Septimus, looking up, they are signaling to me" (*MD* 21). He finds sinister meanings in the words of Shakespeare: "This was now

---

[4] Though Quentin Bells cites Woolf's belief that people laughed at her in the streets as evidence of her insanity, Stephen Trombley suggests that this was not evidence of paranoia—that people were actually laughing at her (Trombley 5).

revealed to Septimus; the message hidden in the beauty of words. The secret signal which one generation passes, under disguise, to the next is loathing, hatred, despair" (*MD* 86). While Septimus's delusions are obviously a product of his illness, his paranoid thoughts also reveal a truth learned through the brutality of war: "For the truth is (let her ignore it) that human beings have neither kindness, nor faith, nor charity beyond what serves to increase the pleasure of the moment. They hunt in packs. Their packs scour the desert and vanish screaming into the wilderness. They desert the fallen" (*MD* 87). This misanthropic message is the meaning that Septimus gleans from his traumatic experiences.

Not only does Septimus understand misanthropic truths about humanity, he also has the megalomaniacal delusion that he is the recipient of an important message that must be delivered to the world. Septimus believes he is the "young man who carries in him the greatest message in the world, and is, moreover, the happiest man in the world, and the most miserable" (*MD* 81). As Kay Redfield Jamison explains, "manic individuals usually have inflated self-esteem, as well as a certainty of conviction about the correctness and importance of their ideas" (13). He feverishly scribbles his messages on scraps of paper: "Men must not cut down trees. There is a God. (He noted such revelations on the backs of envelopes.) Change the world. No one kills from hatred. Make it known (he wrote down)" (*MD* 24). Rezia tells us, "The table was full of those writings; about war, about Shakespeare; about great discoveries; how there is no death" (*MD* 137). When he is too excited to write his messages himself, he dictates to Rezia:

> Lately he had become excited suddenly for no reason . . . and waved his hands and cried out that he knew the truth! He knew everything! . . . She wrote it down just as he spoke it. Some things were very beautiful; others sheer nonsense. And he was always stopping in the middle, changing his mind; wanting to add something; hearing something new; listening with his hand up. (*MD* 137)

Septimus's megalomaniacal delusions, as well as the rapidity and fluidity of his thoughts, are manifestations of severe mania.

In cases of severe mania, religious delusions and megalomania often go hand-in-hand. This is certainly true of Septimus, who believes himself to be the sacrificial lamb of humanity: "Look the unseen bade him, the voice which now communicated with him who was the greatest of mankind, Septimus, lately taken from life to death, the Lord who had come to renew society . . . suffering for ever, the scapegoat, the eternal sufferer" (*MD* 25). Septimus sees himself as a Christ-figure, believing that "it was decreed that he, Septimus, the *lord* of men, should be free; alone . . . he, Septimus, was alone, called forth in advance of the mass of men to hear the truth, to learn the meaning" (*MD* 66; emphasis mine). Septimus believes that it is his duty to deliver this message and the sins of the world, but the only way he can do this is by sacrificing himself: "The whole world was clamouring: Kill yourself, kill yourself, for our sakes" (*MD* 90). In "The Prime Minister," Septimus's delusions of martyrdom are even more elaborate, as he envisions his body as the Eucharist: "One might give one's body to be eaten by the starving, and then, thought Septimus, be a martyr. . . . I shall be immortal, he thought, my name will be on all the placards" (*PM* 586). While the Septimus of *Mrs. Dalloway* doesn't go so far as to say, "He was some sort of Christ probably" (*PM* 585), Septimus does see his suicide as a sacrifice he makes for humanity.

Septimus's suicide, like so many other aspects of his character, is modeled after one of Woolf's experiences. One of her mental breakdowns occurred in 1904 following the death of her father. According to Quentin Bell, "She threw herself from a window, which, however, was not high enough from the ground to cause serious harm. It was here too that she lay in bed, listening to the birds singing in Greek and imagining that King Edward lurked in the azaleas using the foulest possible language" (1: 90). Woolf recreated this experience of madness through the character of Septimus, who also hears birds speaking in Greek: "A sparrow perched on the railing opposite chirped Septimus, Septimus, four or five times over and went on, drawing its notes out, to sing freshly and piercingly in Greek" (*MD* 24). Furthermore, Septimus' fixation on the prime minister reflects Woolf's delusions associated with King Edward. Clearly Septimus served as an outlet through which Woolf could portray her more severe experiences of mental illness.

From the time of Woolf's first breakdown after the death of her mother in 1895 until her own death in 1941, various doctors were called in to treat her. The doctor who treated Woolf during some of her most severe breakdowns was Sir George Savage. The author of *Insanity and Allied Neuroses*—a popular textbook—and the editor of the *Journal of Mental Science*, Savage was one of the most eminent physicians of his day. In Savage's book, he suggests that education for a woman can lead to insanity. His treatment for Woolf consisted of "food, rest and the avoidance of intellectual stimulation" (Trombley 139). Sometimes Savage sent Woolf to a rest home for treatment, while at other times he just prescribed her removal from London and a sleeping draught.[5] Woolf's letters reflect her contemptuous attitude about his methods. When he prescribed the "rest cure" and banished her from London in 1904, she wrote: "I have never spent such a wretched 8 months in my life. And yet that tyrannical, and as I think, shortsighted Savage insists on another two. . . . As a matter of fact my sleep hasn't improved a scrap since I have been here, and his sleeping draught gives me a headache, and nothing else" (*Letters*: 1, 147). When he finally lets her return to London, she writes: "I am feeling really quiet and happy. . . . If only that pigheaded Savage will see that this is the sober truth" (*Letters*: 1,153). Indeed, Savage was quite "pigheaded" in his methods—using the "force of reason" to bully his patients into conforming to his expectations (Trombley 149-52).

After Savage, the other physician primarily responsible for Woolf's treatment was Sir Maurice Craig. Like Savage, Craig was very influential in the field of mental health. He held many key positions, including President of the Psychiatry Section of the Royal Society of Medicine, Chairman of the National Council for Mental Hygiene, and Vice-President of the International Committee for Mental Hygiene. In addition, his *Psychological Medicine* was a popular textbook. Craig's treatment plan doesn't appear to differ significantly from Savage's: "Craig's treatment seems to have consisted in getting his patient to rest, take sleeping draughts, and eat more than was probably good for her" (Trombley 185). Under his guidance, Woolf gained about sixty pounds in two years (Trombley 186). Like Savage, Craig stressed conformity. Trombley explains: "In his diagnosis of madness, symptoms such as delusions, hallucinations, and other morbid phenomena play only a secondary role in determining who is mad and who is sane. The main criterion is always the patient's ability to conform to social expectations" (193).

Just as Woolf recreated her experiences with mental illness in *Mrs. Dalloway*, she also used her own experiences with the doctors who treated her as a basis for Septimus's encounters with Holmes and Sir William Bradshaw. Woolf is critical of both the attitudes and the methods of these doctors. Septimus's attempts to make meaning of his illness have repeatedly been thwarted by Dr. Holmes, who always said "there was nothing the matter with him" (*MD* 23). By denying Septimus's illness, Holmes denies

---

[5] In his writings Savage is critical of drugs—reporting that they can cause paralysis, collapse, inability to read, depression, confusion, hallucinations, dry throat, appetite failure, delusions of persecution—but he gave Virginia sleeping draughts, and she got the veronal for one suicide attempt through him. As Stephen Trombley notes, many of the side-effects that Savage lists are alleged symptoms of insanity that Virginia exhibited (142).

him the chance to recover. Learning that he suffered from shell-shock and that his condition was a normal response to trauma would have been therapeutic in and of itself. This knowledge would have helped Septimus feel that he was not alone and that others understood the reason for his suffering. Holmes denies Septimus this comfort. By denying Septimus a reason for his illness, Holmes makes him feel ashamed and exacerbates his feelings of guilt: "So there was no excuse; nothing whatever the matter, except the sin for which human nature had condemned him to death; that he did not feel" (*MD* 89). In addition to depriving Septimus of a diagnosis and, therefore, a reason for his illness, Holmes belittles his suffering by calling it a "funk" (*MD* 89). Furthermore, Holmes tries to shame Septimus out of his depression by telling him that talk of suicide gave his wife "a very odd idea of English husbands," and asking, "didn't one owe perhaps a duty to one's wife?" (*MD* 90). As Septimus's suicide makes clear, shaming a victim of trauma does not aid the recovery process.

While Holmes continually asserts that there is nothing the matter with Septimus, he dispenses quite a bit of useless advice. Holmes tells Septimus to "take an interest in things outside himself" (*MD* 21) and to "notice real things, go to a music hall, play cricket—that was the very game, Dr. Holmes said" (*MD* 25). In short, Holmes advises Septimus to ignore his illness and conform to society. Such a course of action makes recovery impossible. Moreover, Holmes prescribes "two tabloids of bromide dissolved into a glass of water at bedtime" (*MD* 88). Since bromide is a sedative, it can cause depression to spiral out of control.[6]

Although Holmes says nothing is wrong with Septimus, Sir William Bradshaw "was certain directly he saw the man; it was a case of extreme gravity. It was a case of complete breakdown, with every symptom in an advanced stage" (*MD* 93). Bradshaw regrets that Holmes has been treating Septimus for six weeks, as "[i]t took half his time to undo [those general practitioners'] blunders. Some were irreparable" (*MD* 93). Bradshaw is at least able to diagnose his patient with shell-shock. However, while he never has the chance to treat Septimus, Woolf suggests that Bradshaw's method of treatment would have been unsuccessful as well. Like Holmes, Bradshaw encourages Septimus to "Try to think as little about yourself as possible" (*MD* 96) and conform. Bradshaw is a proponent of the "rest cure," and as such his course of action is to "invoke proportion; order rest in bed; rest in solitude; silence and rest; rest without friends, without books, without messages; six months' rest; until a man who went in

[6] In his memoir about depression, William Styron tells of a similar situation that almost led to his own suicide, when "an insouciant doctor had prescribed [a sedative] as a bedtime aid, telling me airily that I could take it as casually as aspirin" (49).

weighing seven stones six comes out weighing twelve" (*MD* 97). Though many patients reported favorable results from such a cure, Karen DeMeester explains why it is not the proper treatment for victims of trauma: "although it removes sources of agitation or stress that might aggravate individual symptoms, it fails to address the origin of the disorder—the patient's frustrated search for meaning" (87).

In addition to withholding meaning from the patient, the rest cure deprives the patient of the sense of autonomy that is crucial for recovery from trauma. Sir William's treatment largely consists of imposing his will on his patients: "Naked, defenseless, the exhausted, the friendless received the impress of Sir William's will. He swooped; he devoured. He shut people up" (*MD* 99). By imposing his will onto his patients, Bradshaw violates "the cardinal principal of empowering the survivor" (Herman 164). Moreover, by separating patients from their loved ones, Bradshaw deprives them of the emotional support necessary for recovery (Herman 162). Septimus scoffs at the orders of these doctors, "who different in their verdicts (for Holmes said one thing, Bradshaw another), yet judges they were; who mixed the vision and the sideboard; saw nothing clear, yet ruled, yet inflicted. 'Must' they said" (*MD* 145). Septimus's suicide is an act of defiance, as he refuses to surrender his autonomy. Clarissa correctly interprets Septimus's death as a rebellious expression of free will, for he thwarts Bradshaw's "indescribable outrage—forcing your soul" (*MD* 180).

Like Septimus, Woolf was never fully able to exorcise the demons that haunted her. They were always lurking beneath the surface, waiting for a stressful event to trigger their release. By March of 1941, Woolf's anxiety had reached a fever pitch. Her nerves were constantly under attack from the war, as she could always "see a low-flying plane with enemy markings, hear the pop-pop-pop of cannon-fire, the disconcerting noise of bullets ripping the air, the whistle crash of bombs" (Bell 2: 217).[7] In addition, she had just finished *Between the Acts* and was experiencing the usual upheaval of emotions that accompanied the completion of a novel. The combined stress of the novel and the war triggered another breakdown, as the voices within her head unleashed themselves one last time. In her suicide note, Woolf wrote: "I feel certain I am going mad again. I feel we can't go through another of those terrible times. And I shan't recover this time. I begin to hear voices, and I can't concentrate" (qtd. in Bell 2: 226). Confronted with the loss of her autonomy and her mind, Woolf decided to rid herself of her

[7] Both Virginia and Leonard Woolf were in Hitler's Black Book, which listed the names of prominent figures to be immediately arrested and handed over to the Gestapo upon a Nazi invasion of Great Britain.

demons the only way she knew how—by drowning herself in the River Ouse.

Though Woolf ultimately committed suicide, documenting her experiences with trauma and mental illness must have been therapeutic. However, her work was not only a form of therapy that allowed her to cope with madness. In writing *Mrs. Dalloway*, Woolf publicly indicted both the attitudes and treatments of her doctors. She explained to a friend: "It was a subject that I have kept cooling in my mind until I felt I could touch it without bursting into flame all over. You can't think what a raging furnace it is still to me—madness and doctors and being forced" (*Letters* 3: 180). Virginia Woolf refused to assume the role of passive victim that her doctors tried to force upon her. Instead, she took up the pen and actively protested how mad doctors responded to and treated patients suffering from mental illness.

CONCLUSION

Various scholars have noted the association between women and mental illness that has existed in popular cultural for centuries. In the Victorian and Modern eras, that association is clearly demonstrated by gendered theories and categories of mental illness. Both theories of mental illness, like the "reflex theory" of disease causation, and disease categories, such as hysteria, enshrined the cultural association between women and mental illness as a scientific fact. Thus, medical science was used to validate societal beliefs. Like these theories and disease categories, the visual art of the time—particularly the Pre-Raphaelite obsession with Ophelia—both reflected and encouraged the cultural association between women and madness. Scholars have offered various interpretations to explain the cultural association between women and mental illness in the nineteenth and early twentieth centuries. Some have argued that women were driven insane by their repressive gender roles, while others have suggested that the label of "insanity" was applied to rebellious women as a means of punishment. Individual cases lend credence to each of these explanations.

Unfortunately, the association between women and mental illness is not relegated to the past. As Elaine Showalter has observed, "new treatments of mental illness and deinstitutionalization seem to have little effect on the cultural image of women as mental patients" (*Female* 249). The categories of mental illness have changed, but women are still more likely to be treated for mental illnesses. Women are twice as likely to be diagnosed with depression as men (World Health Organization). And according to Judith Herman, a professor of clinical psychiatry at Harvard Medical School and one of the world's foremost authorities on trauma, "the most common post-traumatic disorders are not those of men in war but of women in civilian life" (28). Moreover, women are more likely to be disabled by mental illness than men: "The disability associated with mental illness falls most heavily on those who experience three or more comorbid disorders. Again, women predominate" (World Health Organization). As in the past, it is impossible to determine whether women actually suffer from mental illnesses more than men, or whether they just appear to suffer from mental illness more because of a bias in diagnosis. However, a bias does exist: "Doctors are more likely to diagnose depression in women compared with men, even when they have similar scores on standardized measures of depression or present with identical symptoms" (World Health Organization). Not only is there a gender bias in diagnosing mental illness, there is a bias in the treatment of mental illness. According to the World Health Organization, "Female gender is a significant predictor of being prescribed mood altering psychotropic drugs." As Showalter has noted, "[i]n contemporary practice, medical management has replaced moral management as a way of containing women's suffering without confronting its causes" (*Female* 249).

In the last lines of *The Female Malady,* Showalter suggests that women need to speak up for themselves in order to overturn the cultural association between women and mental illness and rid the treatment of mental health of misogyny:

> Throughout the history of psychiatry, there have been many male liberators—Pinel, Conolly, Charcot, Freud, Laing—who claimed to free madwomen from the chains of their confinement to obtuse and misogynistic medical practice. Yet when women are spoken for but do not speak for themselves, such dramas of liberation become only the opening scenes of the next drama of confinement. Until women break them for themselves, the chains that make madness a female malady, like Blake's 'mind-forg'd manacles,' will simply forge themselves anew. (*Female* 250)

By implying that women have not historically spoken up for themselves, Showalter perpetuates the image of the female mental patient as a silent victim. Unfortunately, she is not alone. Since the 1980s, various scholars have studied the cultural association between women and mental illness. However, these studies typically portray female mental patients as victims, much as Wilkie Collins did a century and a half ago. As this book has attempted to show, that image is a distortion of the truth. Throughout the Victorian and Modern eras, some women refused to silently submit to the diagnoses and treatments that male doctors tried to force upon them. They were active protestors, not silent victims, of the misogynist medical diagnoses and practices that affected their lives.

Many women who believed they had been inaccurately diagnosed as insane and locked in asylums wrote narratives detailing their experiences. The authors of these asylum narratives frequently suggested that the label of "madness" was used as a punishment against them as women who defied social conventions. Indeed, mental illness was virtually synonymous with non-conformity for men and women alike. However, female non-conformists were particularly vulnerable to institutionalization because the cultural association between women and madness made some doctors quick to diagnose women as mentally ill.

The public was aware of the unwarranted confinement of some mental patients. In England, this led to a series of lunacy panics and the publication of novels such as Mary Elizabeth Braddon's *Lady Audley's Secret* (1862) and *The Woman in White* (1860) by Wilkie Collins. While Collins sympathizes with the plight of women who have been punished with incarceration in insane asylums, his novel portrays these women as mentally weak and helpless victims who need to be saved and guided by men. Mary Elizabeth Braddon, on the other hand, portrays the punishment of deviant women as a necessary measure to ensure the safety of society.

Many people in the Victorian and early Modern periods believed they had a duty to incarcerate—and sometimes rehabilitate—deviants. Rehabilitation often involved forcing patients to conform through "moral management" and the enforced passivity of the "rest cure." By protesting their institutionalization and fighting for their rights, many women refused to conform to society's views of appropriate behavior for women. Mary Lincoln was one such woman, but while she campaigned for her rights as an individual, many women campaigned for the rights of others as well.

Because these women had been wrongfully institutionalized themselves, they campaigned to change the admission laws to insane asylums. These reformers blamed their incarcerations on unfair gender biases, and they fought to advance woman's rights. As Sylvia Hoffert explains, "[p]ersonal circumstances determined which aspects of gender discrimination triggered feminist consciousness and brought individual women into the woman's rights movement" (9). Some advocates were inspired to fight for woman's rights when they experienced discrimination in their temperance, anti-slavery, or church groups. Others were inspired to action after witnessing discrimination in the workplace or in the legal system. The authors of asylum narratives were compelled to struggle for reform by their own unjust incarcerations in insane asylums. In protesting the gender bias that led to their institutionalization, the authors of these narratives employed the rhetoric of natural rights that was a part of the American political tradition established by the Declaration of Independence. They also used the metaphor of slavery to describe the condition of women in America. Thus, they utilized the discourse that woman's rights advocates established to protest their grievances and sway public opinion in their favor (see Hoffert).

While the authors of these asylum narratives were concerned with improving the lives of women, they were also humanitarians concerned with improving the lives of the insane—men and women alike—who were vulnerable to abuse and could not stand up for themselves. As Jeffrey Geller and Maxine Harris explain, these "women clearly wrote in the reform tradition of the turn of the century; they intended that their experiences be used to assist the efforts to improve conditions within asylums and to change the laws that kept men and women incarcerated against their will" (5). Asylum narratives prompted "a drive to secure legislation that would effectively guard the rights of patients and circumscribe the powers of hospital officials," as well as "an increase in the number of legislative investigations into the internal activities of mental hospitals and the alleged abuses of patients" (Grob 264-65).

The most famous and influential of these patients turned reformers was Elizabeth Packard. For thirty years after her release in 1863, Packard strove to change asylum laws around the country (Himelhoch and Shaffer 345). Packard travelled from state to state in her reform efforts, and her methods were systematic. When she first arrived in a state, Packard travelled from town to town selling her books. Next, she sought the support of influential people and legislators for the bill she planned to introduce. Then Packard hired a local lawyer to draw up her bill and present it to the legislature. As the bill was being debated, she campaigned for it by distributing handbills and advertising it in local newspapers (Himelhoch and Shaffer 369). Using these methods, Packard inspired asylum reform around the country. She introduced three types of bills, each with a different objective:

> (1) to keep sane people out of mental institutions by tightening up commitment procedures and narrowing the definition of mental illness, (2) to obtain effective outside supervision of asylum managers in order to guarantee humane treatment of the patients, and (3) to protect the postal rights of patients as an added safeguard against unjust confinement and bad treatment. (Himelhoch and Shaffer 371-72)

In addition to the laws governing insane asylums, Packard also campaigned for the property rights of married women. According to her obituary in the *Chicago Tribune*, her reform activities led to the passage of thirty-four bills in various states. Another newspaper proclaimed, "no woman of her day, except possibly Harriet Beecher Stowe, exerted a wider influence in the interest of humanity" (qtd. in Himelhoch and Shaffer 374).

Many scholars—such as Lori Ginzberg and Carolyn Lawes—have devoted their attention to female reformers in the nineteenth century. However, the asylum reform movement has not been interpreted as a feminist movement. In fact, the asylum reform movement in America is generally understudied. When scholars address asylum reform in America, they tend to focus on one woman's struggle within the movement. Some scholars—such as David Gollaher and David Lightner—have examined Dorothea Dix's labors to improve asylum conditions, while others—such as Jennifer Levison and Barbara Sapinsley—have described Elizabeth Packard's struggle to change admission laws. However, by focusing on one woman's efforts these historians risk turning a broader movement into a one-woman crusade. By comparing the work of various reformers struggling to change asylum laws and conditions, it becomes clear that the efforts of Packard and Dix are part of a larger movement that was driven by women. The struggle for asylum reform was a feminist movement in pursuit of social justice, and it was largely a movement composed of women who had been unjustly institutionalized themselves.

Although the cultural association between women and madness allowed many women to be wrongfully confined in the Victorian and Modern periods, this is not to say that no women suffered from mental illness. Both Charlotte Perkins Gilman and Virginia Woolf acknowledged that they suffered from bouts of mental illness, and they wrote about their illnesses and the treatments they received in both fictional and non-fictional forms. Writing about such an experience was probably therapeutic, but it was also an act of protest. Gilman and Woolf both sought medical treatment for their illness, and both disapproved of the treatment they received. They were treated with the "rest cure," which enforced passivity on the patient. While some patients reportedly improved under this treatment, Gilman and Woolf disparaged the "rest cure." Neither woman wanted to be forced into playing the role of the passive female. Like the authors of asylum narratives, Gilman and Woolf rejected the role of the silent and submissive woman and assumed the active role of publicly protesting aspects of mental healthcare. Both women protested attitudes towards mental illness expressed by doctors and the public at large, and they critiqued treatments offered by the medical community.

The categories and theories of mental illness in the Victorian and Modern periods attest to the connection between women and madness that existed in the public imagination. This connection is reflected in the Pre-Raphaelite obsession with Ophelia, the madwoman who had the honor of being the most depicted subject in nineteenth-century British art. By constantly presenting the figure of the madwoman to the public, the Pre-Raphaelites actually helped perpetuate the cultural association between women and madness. This cultural association was not just generally demeaning to women; it also had significant ramifications in the lives of many individuals. As the asylum narratives and the case of Mary Lincoln illustrate, the cultural association between women and madness made it easier for many women to be labeled "mad" and confined in insane asylums. The public was aware that sometimes women were punished for rebelling against social conventions through institutionalization, as both *Lady Audley's Secret* and *The Woman in White* demonstrate. While some sympathized with such women, others saw them as justly punished for their deviancy. As part of their punishment, these rebellious women were often subjected to treatments that were designed to enforce conformity. Even some women like Charlotte Perkins Gilman and Virginia Woolf, who sought treatment for mental illness, protested the "rest cure" that demanded silence and submission from the patient. The authors of asylum narratives, Mary Lincoln, Charlotte Perkins Gilman, and Virginia Woolf all refused to assume the role of passive victim. Instead, they assumed an active role by protesting the laws, diagnoses, and treatments that had a negative impact on their lives.

BIBLIOGRAPHY

Abelson, Elaine S. "The Invention of Kleptomania." *Signs* 15.1 (1989): 123-43. *JSTOR*. Web. 24 Jan 2013.

Appignanesi, Lisa. *Mad, Bad, and Sad: A History of Women and the Mind Doctors*. New York: Norton, 2008. Print.

Baker, Jean H. *Mary Todd Lincoln: A Biography*. New York: Norton, 1987. Print.

Bederman, Gail. "'Not to Sex—But to Race!' Charlotte Perkins Gilman, Civilized Anglo-Saxon Womanhood, and the Return of the Primitive Rapist." *Manliness and Civilization: A Cultural History of Gender and Race in the United States, 1880-1917.* Chicago: U of Chicago P, 1995. 121-69. Print.

Bell, Quentin. *Virginia Woolf: A Biography*. 2 vols. New York: Harcourt, 1972. Print.

Berry, Stephen. *House of Abraham: Lincoln and the Todds, a Family Divided by War*. Boston: Houghton Mifflin, 2007. Print.

Birnbaum, Michele. "Racial Hysteria: Female Pathology and Race Politics in Frances Harper's *Iola Leroy* and W. D. Howell's *An Imperative Duty*." *African American Review* 33.1 (1999): 7-23. *EBSCO*. Web. 6 Oct. 2011.

Braddon, Mary Elizabeth. 1862. *Lady Audley's Secret*. New York: Dover, 1974. Print.

Bradwell, James B. Letter to Dr. R. J. Patterson. 19 Aug. 1875. Emerson, *Insanity Case* 119.

Bradwell, Myra. Letter to Elizabeth Edwards. 11 Aug. 1875. Emerson, *Insanity Case* 109.

Braude, Ann. *Radical Spirits: Spiritualism and Women's Rights in Nineteenth-Century America*. 2nd ed. Bloomington: Indiana UP, 2001. Print.

Briggs, Laura. "The Race of Hysteria: 'Overcivilization' and the 'Savage' Woman in Late Nineteenth-Century Obstetrics and Gynecology." *American Quarterly* 52.2 (2000): 246-73. *JSTOR*. Web. 6 Oct. 2011.

Brincklé, Adriana P. "Life Among the Insane." *North American Review* 144 (1887): 190-99. *Google Books*. Web. 22 Mar. 2011.

Brokoph-Mauch, Gudrun. "Salome and Ophelia: The Portrayal of Women in Art and Literature at the Turn of the Century." *The Turn of the Century: Modernism and Modernity in Literature and the Arts*. Eds. Christian Berg, Frank Direux, and Geert Lernout. Berlin: de Gruyter, 1995. 466-74. Print.

Burlingame, Michael. *The Inner World of Abraham Lincoln*. Urbana: U of Illinois P, 1994.

Chesler, Phyllis. Foreword. Gellar and Harris.

Clinton, Catherine. *Mrs. Lincoln: A Life*. New York: Harper, 2009. Print.

"Clouded Reason." Emerson, *Insanity Case* 15-22. Rpt. of *Chicago Tribune* 20 May 1875.

Collins, Wilkie. Preface. 1860. *The Woman in White*. 1861. Oxford: Oxford UP, 1996. Print.

—. *The Woman in White*. 1861. Oxford: Oxford UP, 1996. Print.

Cottier, Lizzie D. "Preface." *The Right Spirit*. Buffalo, NY: Courier, 1885. 5-14. *Google Books*. Web. 19 Apr. 2011.

Cox, Robert S. *Body and Soul: A Sympathetic History of American Spiritualism*. Charlottesville: U of Virginia P, 2003. Print.

Crabtree, Adam. *From Mesmer to Freud: Magnetic Sleep and the Roots of Psychological Healing*. New Haven: Yale UP, 1993. Print.

Cramer, Patricia Morgne. "Trauma and Lesbian Returns in Virginia Woolf's *The Voyage Out* and *The Years*." *Virginia Woolf and Trauma:*

Embodied Texts. Eds. Suzette Henke and David Eberly. New York: Pace UP, 2007. 19-50. Print.

Currie, Richard A. "*All the Year Round* and the State of Victorian Psychiatry." *Dickens Quarterly* 12.1 (1995): 18-24. Print.

Davis, Phebe B. *Two Years and Three Months in the New York Lunatic Asylum at Utica; Together with the Outlines of Twenty Years' Peregrinations in Syracuse*. 1855. Geller and Harris 47-57.

DeMeester, Karen. "Trauma, Post-Traumatic Stress Disorder, and Obstacles to Postwar Recovery in *Mrs. Dalloway*." *Virginia Woolf and Trauma*. Eds. Suzette Henke and David Eberly. New York: Pace UP, 2007. 77-93. Print.

Dijkstra, Bram. *Idols of Perversity*. New York: Oxford UP, 1986. Print.

Dock, Julie Bates, Daphne Ryan Allen, Jennifer Palais, and Kristen Tracy. "'But One Expects That': Charlotte Perkins Gilman's 'The Yellow Wallpaper' and the Shifting Light of Scholarship." *PMLA* 111 (1996): 52-65. *JSTOR*. Web. 21 Mar 14.

Donaldson, Norman. Introduction. Braddon v-xiv.

Donaldson, Sandra M. "'Ophelia' in Elizabeth Siddal Rossetti's Poem 'A Year and a Day.'" *The Journal of Pre-Raphaelite Studies* 2.1 (1981): 127-33. Print.

Drake, Daniel. "Diseases of the Negro Population." *Southern Medical and Surgical Journal* 2 (1845): 341-43. *Google Books*. Web. 21 Nov. 2011.

Edwards, Elizabeth. Letter to Myra Bradwell. 3 Aug. 1875. Emerson, *Insanity Case* 98.

—. Letter to Robert Lincoln. 15 Sep. 1875. Emerson, *Insanity Case* 145-46.

—. Letter to Robert Lincoln. 5 Nov. 1875. Emerson, *Insanity Case* 147-48.

Edwards, Ninian. Letter to Robert Lincoln. 17 Nov. 1875. Emerson, *Insanity Case* 155.

—. Letter to Robert Lincoln. 14 Jan. 1876. Emerson, *Insanity Case* 167.

—. Letter to Robert Lincoln. 17 June 1876. Emerson, *Insanity Case* 185.

Emerson, Jason. *The Madness of Mary Lincoln*. Carbondale: Southern Illinois UP, 2007. Print.

—. *Mary Lincoln's Insanity Case: A Documentary History*. Urbana: University of Illinois UP, 2012. Print.

Faraci, Mary. "Imagining Ophelia in Christina Rossetti's 'Sleeping at Last.'" *Victorian Newsletter* 111 (2007): 8-9. Print.

Foucault, Michel. *History of Madness.* Ed. Jean Khalfa. Trans. Jonathan Murphy and Jean Khalfa. London: Routledge, 2006. Print.

Gellar, Jeffrey L. and Maxine Harris, eds. *Women of the Asylum: Voices from behind the Walls, 1840-1945*. New York: Doubleday, 1995. Print.

Gilbert, Pamela K. "Madness and Civilization: Generic Opposition in Mary Elizabeth Braddon's *Lady Audley's Secret*." *Essays in Literature* 23.2 (1996): 218-33. Print.

Gilman, Charlotte Perkins. Letter to S. Weir Mitchell. 19 Apr. 1887. Rpt. in Knight. 271-74.

—. *The Living of Charlotte Perkins Gilman: An Autobiography*. Madison: U of Wisconsin P, 1935. Print.

—. "The 'Nervous Breakdown' of Women." *Forerunner* 7 (1916): 202-06. *Radical Periodicals in the United States, 1890-1960.* New York: Greenwood Reprint Corp, 1968. *Hathi Trust Digital Library*. Web. 21 Mar. 2014.

—. "The Yellow Wallpaper." 1892. *"The Yellow Wallpaper" and Other Writings.* New York: Random House, 2000. 3-20. Print.

—. "Why I Wrote *The Yellow Wallpaper*." 1913. *National Library of Medicine*. Web. 28 Apr. 2011.

Ginzberg, Lori D. *Women and the Work of Benevolence: Morality, Politics, and Class in the Nineteenth-Century United States*. New Haven: Yale UP, 1990. Print.

Gollaher, David. *Voice for the Mad: The Life of Dorothea Dix*. New York: Free Press, 1995. Print.

Grob, Gerald. *Mental Institutions in America: Social Policy to 1875*. New York: Free Press, 1973. Print.

Hawksley, Lucinda. *Lizzie Siddal: Face of the Pre-Raphaelites*. New York: Walker, 2004. Print.

Henke, Suzette A. *Shattered Subjects: Trauma and Testimony in Women's Life-Writing*. New York: St. Martin's, 2000. Print.

Herman, Judith Lewis. *Trauma and Recovery: The Aftermath of Violence—from Domestic Abuse to Political Terror*. New York: Basic Books, 1992. Print.

Herndon, William H., and Jesse W. Weik. *Herndon's Lincoln; The True Story of a Great Life: The History and Personal Recollections of Abraham Lincoln*. 1889. Eds. Douglas L. Wilson and Rodney O. Davis. Urbana: U of Illinois P, 2006. Print.

Himelhoch, Myra Samuels, and Arthur H. Shaffer. "Elizabeth Packard: Nineteenth-Century Crusader for the Rights of Mental Patients." *Journal of American Studies* 13.3 (1979): 343-75. *JSTOR*. Web. 5 May 2013.

Hoffert, Sylvia D. *When Hens Crow: The Woman's Rights Movement in Antebellum America*. Bloomington: Indiana UP, 1995. Print.

Hubert, Susan J. *Questions of Power: The Politics of Women's Madness Narratives*. Newark: U of Delaware P, 2002. Print.

Huffels, Natalie. "Tracing Traumatic Memory in *The Woman in White*: Psychic Shock, Victorian Science, and the Narrative Strategy of the Shadow-*Bildungsroman*." *Victorian Review* 37.1 (2011): 42-61. *Project Muse*. Web. 15 Jan. 2014.

Hyder, C.K. "Wilkie Collins and the *Woman in White*." *PMLA* 54 (1939): 297-303. *JSTOR*. Web. 01 Oct. 2014.

Jamison, Kay Redfield. *Touched with Fire: Manic-Depressive Illness and the Artistic Temperament*. New York: Free Press, 1993. Print.

Janet, Pierre. *The Major Symptoms of Hysteria*. 2nd ed. New York: Macmillan, 1924. Print.

Kiefer, Carol Soloman, ed. *The Myth and Madness of Ophelia*. Amherst: Mead Art Museum, 2001. Print.

Klein, Herbert G. "Strong Women and Feeble Men: Upsetting Gender Stereotypes in Mary Elizabeth Braddon's *Lady Audley's Secret*." *Atenea* 28.1 (2008): 161-74. Print.

Knight, Denise D. "'All the Facts of the Case': Gilman's Lost Letter to Dr. S. Weir Mitchell." *American Literary Realism* 37 (2005): 259-77. *JSTOR*. 21 Mar. 2014. Web.

Kurata, Marilyn. "Wrongful Confinement: The Betrayal of Women by Men, Medicine, and Law." *Victorian Scandals: Representations of Gender and Class*. Ed. Kristine Ottesen Garrigan. Athens: Ohio UP, 1992. 43-68. Print.

Lake, Caroline E. "Testimony of Mrs. Caroline E. Lake, of Aurora, Ill." Vol. 2 of Packard, *The Prisoner's Hidden Life* 140-42.

Lathrop, Clarissa Caldwell. *A Secret Institution.* 1890. Geller and Harris 152-60. Print.

Carolyn J. Lawes. *Women and Reform in a New England Community, 1815-1860*. Lexington: UP of Kentucky, 2000. Print.

Leavitt, Judith Walzer. "Under the Shadow of Maternity: American Women's Responses to Death and Debility Fears in Nineteenth-Century Childbirth." *Women and Health in America: Historical Readings.* Madison: U of Wisconsin P, 1999. 328-46. Print.

Leavy, Barbara Fass. "Wilkie Collins's Cinderella: The History of Psychology and *The Woman in White*." *Dickens Study Annual* 10 (1982): 91-141. Print.

Lee, Kate. *A Year at Elgin Insane Asylum*. 1902. Gellar and Harris 203-13. Print.

Levison, Jennifer Rebecca. "Elizabeth Parsons Ware Packard: An Advocate for Cultural, Religious, and Legal Change." *Alabama Law Review* 54.3 (2003): 985-1075. *Alabama Law Review*. Web. 3 Oct. 2011.

Lincoln, Robert. Letter to David Davis. 16 Nov. 1875. Emerson, *Insanity Case* 153-55.

—. Letter to Elizabeth Edwards. 7 Aug. 1875. Emerson, *Insanity Case* 102-05.

—. Letter to Henry T. Blow. 4 Aug. 1875. Emerson, *Insanity Case* 99-101.

—. Letter to Ninian Edwards. 21 Dec. 1875. Emerson, *Insanity Case* 162-63.

Lightner, David L., ed. *Asylum, Prison, and Poorhouse: The Writings and Reform Work of Dorothea Dix in Illinois*. Carbondale, Illinois: Southern Illinois UP, 1999. Print.

Lunt, Adeline T. P. *Behind Bars*. New York: Lee, Shepard, and Dillingham, 1871. *Open Library*. Web. 31 Mar. 2011.

Lytton, Rosina Bulwer. *A Blighted Life: A True Story*. 1880. Bristol: Thoemmes, 1996. Print.

Marsh, Jan. *Elizabeth Siddal, 1829-1862: Pre-Raphaelite Artist*. Sheffield: Ruskin Gallery, 1991. Print.

—. *Pre-Raphaelite Women: Images of Femininity*. New York: Harmony Books, 1988. Print.

Marsh, Jan, and Pamela Gerrish Nunn. *Women Artists and the Pre-Raphaelite Movement*. London: Virago, 1989. Print.

Matus, Jill L. "Disclosure as 'Cover-up': The Discourse of Madness in *Lady Audley's Secret*." *University of Toronto Quarterly* 62.3 (1993): 334-55. Print.

McCandless, Peter. "Liberty and Lunacy: Victorians and Wrongful Confinement." *Madhouse, Mad-Doctors, and Madmen*. Ed. Andrew Scull. Philadelphia: U of Pennsylvania P, 1981. 339-62. Print.

McGarry, Molly. *Ghosts of Futures Past: Spiritualism and the Cultural Politics of Nineteenth-Century America*. Berkeley: U of California P, 2008. Print.

Metcalf, Ada. *Lunatic Asylums: and How I Became an Inmate of One. Doctors, Incidents, Humbuggery*. 1876. Geller and Harris 124-31.

Micale, Mark S. *Approaching Hysteria: Disease and Its Interpretations*. Princeton: Princeton UP, 1995. Print.

Miller, D.A. "Cage Aux Folles: Sensation and Gender in Wilkie Collins's *The Woman in White*." *Representations* 14 (1986): 107-36. Print.

Minard, Sarah. "The Testimony of Mrs. Sarah Minard, of St. Charles, Ill." Vol. 2 of Packard, *The Prisoner's Hidden Life* 126-31.

Mitchell, Silas Weir. *Doctor and Patient.* Philadelphia: Lippincott, 1888. *Google Books*. Web. 22 Mar. 2014.

—. *Fat and Blood: An Essay on the Treatment of Certain Forms of Neurasthenia and Hysteria*. 4th ed. London: Lippincott, 1885. *Google Books*. Web. 28 Apr. 2011.

Morrow, Honoré Wilsie. *Mary Todd Lincoln; An Appreciation of the Wife of Abraham Lincoln*. New York: Morrow, 1928. Print.

"Mrs. Lincoln: She is Recovering from Her Mental Malady." Emerson, *Insanity Case* 120-22. Rpt. of *Chicago Post and Mail* 21 Aug. 1875.

"Mrs. Lincoln: A Startling Interview upon Her Case with Judge Bradwell." Emerson, *Insanity Case* 123-25. Rpt. of *Chicago Post and Mail* 23 Aug. 1875.

"Mrs. Lincoln: A Visit to Her by *The Post and Mail* Correspondent." Emerson, *Insanity Case* 84-90. Rpt. of *Chicago Post and Mail* 13 July 1875.

Neely, Mark E., and R. Gerald McMurtry. *The Insanity File: The Case of Mary Todd Lincoln*. Carbondale: Southern Illinois UP, 1986. Print.

Patterson, R. J. Letter to Myra Bradwell. 9 Aug. 1875. Emerson, *Insanity Case* 107.

Olsen, Sophia N. B. *Mrs. Olsen's Narrative of Her One Year's Imprisonment, at Jacksonville Insane Asylum: With the Testimony of Mrs. Minard, Mrs. Shedd, Mrs. Yates, and Mrs. Lake, All Corroborated by the Investigating Committee of the Legislature of Illinois*. Vol. 2 of Packard, *The Prisoner's Hidden Life* 1-121.

—. "The Prisoner's Song." Vol. 2 of Packard, *The Prisoner's Hidden Life* 122-24.

—. "Spare the Creed!" Vol. 1 of Packard, The Prisoner's Hidden Life 23.

Packard, Elizabeth P. W. *The Exposure on Board the Atlantic and Pacific Car of Emancipation for the Slaves of Old Columbia, Engineered by the Lightening Express; or, Christianity and Calvinism Compared. With an Appeal to the Government to Emancipate the Slaves of the Marriage Union*. Chicago: Clark, 1864. *Hathi Trust Digital Library*. Web. 20 Apr. 2011.

—. *Marital Power Exemplified in Mrs. Packard's Trial, and Self-Defense from the Charge of Insanity; or Three Years' Imprisonment for Religious Belief, by the Arbitrary Will of a Husband, with an Appeal to the Government to so Change the Laws as to Afford Legal Protection to Married Women.* Hartford, CT: Case, Lockwood, & Brainard, 1866. *Google Books*. Web. 26 Feb. 2011.

—. *Modern Persecutions, or Insane Asylums Unveiled, As Demonstrated by the Report of the Investigating Committee of the Legislature of Illinois*. 2 vols. Hartford, CT: Case, Lockwood, & Brainard, 1874. *Internet Archive*. Web. 20 Apr. 2011.

—. *The Prisoner's Hidden Life, or, Insane Asylums Unveiled: As Demonstrated by the Report of the Investigating Committee of the Legislature of Illinois. Together with Mrs. Packard's Coadjutors' Testimony*. 2 vols. Chicago: A.B. Case, 1868. *Internet Archive*. Web. 20 Apr. 2011.

Parlin, Melissa. "Refashioning Cordelia, Ophelia, and Juliet: The Strength of Julia Margaret Cameron's Suffering Women." *Selected Papers of the Ohio Valley Shakespeare Conference* 2 (2008): 30-42. Print.

Pennell, Lemira Clarissa. *This Red Book is Partly a Reprint of What Was Published in 1883, and Later*. 1886. Geller and Harris 147-51.

Peterson, Kaara. "Framing Ophelia: Representation and the Pictorial Tradition." *Mosaic: A Journal for the Interdisciplinary Study of Literature* 31.3 (1998): n.p. *Proquest*. Web. 28 Apr. 2012.

Rhodes, James A., and Dean Jauchius. *The Trial of Mary Todd Lincoln.* Indianapolis: Bobbs-Merrill, 1959. Print.

Roberts, Leonard, and Mary Virginia Evans. "'Sweets to the Sweet': Arthur Hughes's Versions of Ophelia." *The Journal of Pre-Raphaelite Studies* 1.2 (1988): 26-36. Print.

Rossetti, Christina. "Sleeping at Last." *About.com*. Web. 29 Apr. 2012.

Russell, Alice Bingham. *A Plea for the Insane by Friends of the Living Dead*. 1898. Geller and Harris 192-202.

Russett, Cynthia Eagle. *Sexual Science: The Victorian Construction of Womanhood.* Cambridge: Harvard UP, 1989. Print.

"A Sad Revelation." Emerson, *Insanity Case* 22-31. Rpt. of *Chicago Times* 20 May 1875.

Sapinsley, Barbara. *The Private War of Mrs. Packard.* Saint Paul: Paragon House, 1991. Print.

"Scene in a Private Mad-House." *Asylum Journal* 1 (1842): 1. Geller and Harris 1-3. Print.

Scharnhorst, Gary. *Charlotte Perkins Gilman: A Bibliography*. Metuchen, NJ: Scarecrow, 1985. Print.

Scott, Bonnie Kime. Introduction. Woolf, *Mrs. Dalloway* xxxv-lxviii.

Shakespeare, William. *The Tragedy of Hamlet, Prince of Denmark. The Riverside Shakespeare*. 2nd ed. Eds. G. Blakemore Evans and J. J. M. Tobin. Boston: Houghton Mifflin, 1997. 1189-1245. Print.

Shedd, Tirzah F. "Testimony Presented to the Committee by Mrs. Tirzah F. Shedd, of Aurora, Illinois." Vol. 2 of Packard, *The Prisoner's Hidden Life* 132-37.

Showalter, Elaine. *The Female Malady: Women, Madness, and English Culture, 1830-1980*. New York: Pantheon, 1985. Print.

—. "Representing Ophelia: Women, Madness, and the Responsibilities of Feminist Criticism." *Shakespeare and the Question of Theory*. Eds. Patricia Parker and Geoffrey Hartman. New York: Methuen, 1985. 77-94. Print.

Shumaker, Conrad. "'Too Terribly Good to Be Printed': Charlotte Gilman's 'The Yellow Wallpaper.'" *American Literature* 57 (1985): 588-599. *JSTOR*. Web. 21 Mar. 2014.

Siddal, Elizabeth. "A Year and a Day." *PoemHunter.com*. Web. 29 Apr. 2012.

Small, Helen. "'In the Guise of Science': Literature and the Rhetoric of 19th-Century Psychiatry." *History of the Human Sciences* 7.1 (1994): 27-55. Print.

Smith-Rosenberg, Carroll. "From Puberty to Menopause: The Cycle of Femininity in Nineteenth-Century America." *Feminist Studies* 1 (1973): 58-72. Print.

—. "The Hysterical Woman: Sex Roles and Role Conflict in Nineteenth-Century America." *Social Research* 39.4 (1972): 652-78. Print.

Smith-Rosenberg, Carroll, & Charles Rosenberg. "The Female Animal: Medical and Biological Views of Women and Their Role in Nineteenth-Century America." *Journal of American History* 60 (1973): 332–56. Print.

Stanton, Elizabeth Cady. *Eighty Years and More (1815-1897): Reminiscences of Elizabeth Cady Stanton.* New York: European Publishing, 1898. *Google Books*. Web. 15 Mar. 2014.

Stern, Rebecca. "'Personation' and 'Good Marking Ink': Sanity, Performativity, and Biology in Victorian Sensation Fiction." *Nineteenth-Century Studies* 14 (2000): 35-62. Print.

Sucksmith, H.P. Appendix E. "The Main Source of the *Woman in White*." *The Woman in White* by Wilkie Collins. London: 1975. 599-600. Print.

Sutherland, John. Introduction. *The Woman in White*. By Wilkie Collins. Oxford: Oxford UP, 1996. vi-xxiii. Print.

Styron, William. *Darkness Visible: A Memoir of Madness*. New York: Vintage, 1992. Print.

Swett, Leonard. Letter to David Davis. 24 May 1875. Emerson, *Insanity Case* 44-50.

Taylor, Jenny Bourne. "Psychology and Sensation: The Narrative of Moral Management in *The Woman in White*." *Critical Survey* 2.1 (1990): 49-56. Print.

Theriot, Nancy. "Diagnosing Unnatural Motherhood: Nineteenth-Century Physicians and 'Puerperal Insanity.'" *Women and Health in America: Historical Readings*. Madison: U of Wisconsin P, 1999. 405-21. Print.

—. "Negotiating Illness: Doctors, Patients, and Families in the Nineteenth-Century." *Journal of the History of the Behavioral Sciences* 37.4 (2001): 349–368. Print.

—. "Women's Voices in Nineteenth-Century Medical Discourse: A Step toward Deconstructing Science." *Signs* 19.1 (1993): 1-31. Print.

Thrailkill, Jane F. "Doctoring 'The Yellow Wallpaper.'" *ELH* 69 (2002): 525-66. *JSTOR*. Web. 21 Mar. 2014.

Treichler, Paula A. "Escaping the Sentence: Diagnosis and Discourse in 'The Yellow Wallpaper.'" *Tulsa Studies in Women's Literature* 3 (1984): 61-77. *JSTOR*. Web. 21 Mar. 2014.

Trombley, Stephen. *'All that Summer She was Mad': Virginia Woolf and Her Doctors*. London: Junction Books, 1981. Print.

Wheeler, Samuel P. "Solving a Lincoln Literary Mystery: 'Little Eddie.'" *Journal of the Abraham Lincoln Association* 33.2 (2012): 34.36. *University of Michigan.* Web. 3 Apr. 2014.

Wood, Ann Douglas. "'The Fashionable Diseases': Women's Complaints and Their Treatment in Nineteenth-Century America." *The Journal of Interdisciplinary History* 4 (1973): 25-52. *JSTOR*. Web. 21 Mar. 2014.

Woolf, Virginia. *The Diary of Virginia Woolf.* Eds. Anne Olivier Bell with Andrew McNeillie. 4 vols. New York: Harcourt, 1977-82. Print.

—. *Jacob's Room.* 1925. Ed. Mark Hussey. Orlando: Harcourt, 2008. Print.

—. *The Letters of Virginia Woolf.* Eds. Nigel Nicholson and Joanne Trautmann. 6 vols. New York: Harcourt, 1975-1980. Print.

—. *Moments of Being.* Ed. Jeanne Schulkind. 2nd ed. San Diego: Harcourt, 1985. Print.

—. *Mrs. Dalloway.* 1925. Ed. Mark Hussey. New York: Harcourt, 2005. Print.

—. "The Prime Minister." Ed. Suzette Henke. *Gender in Modernism*. Ed. Bonnie Kime Scott. Urbana: U of Illinois P, 2007. 581-87. Print.

—. *To the Lighthouse.* 1927. Ed. Mark Hussey. Orlando: Harcourt, 2005. Print.

—. *The Voyage Out.* San Diego: Harcourt, 1920. Print.

—. *The Waves.* 1931. Ed. Mark Hussey. Orlando: Harcourt, 2006. Print.

—. *The Years.* 1939. Ed. Mark Hussey. Orlando: Harcourt, 2008. Print.

World Health Organization. "Gender Disparities and Women's Health: The Facts." *World Health Organization*. Web. 2 Apr. 2014.

Young, Alan R. "The Ophelia Phenomenon." *Hamlet and the Visual Arts, 1709-1900*. Newark: U of Delaware P, 2002. 279-345. Print.

Ziegler, Georgianna. "Sweet Rose of May: Ophelia through Victorian Eyes." *The Myth and Madness of Ophelia*. Ed. Carol Soloman Kiefer. Amherst: Mead Art Museum, 2001. 41-51. Print.